FABULOUS HEALTH:

A Simple Plan To Get Well And Stay Well

Terri Chrisman

Copyright © 2025 Terri Chrisman FABULOUS HEALTH: A Simple Plan To Get Well And Stay Well. All rights reserved.

The author and the publisher expressly disclaim any liability, loss, or risk which is incurred as a consequence, directly or indirectly, of the use and application of any contents of this work.

ISBN: 979-8-9985783-8-0

Book cover design: Peter Asprey, Asprey Creative
https://www.aspreycreative.com.au

Interior layout: Melanie Mitchell, Overall Productions
https://overallproductionsmm.wixsite.com/

Publisher: Fabulous Health, Dallas, Tx.

The right of Terri Chrisman, identified as the author of this work, has been asserted in accordance with The Copyright Designs and Patents Act 1988.

No part of this work may be reproduced in any material form (including photocopying or storing by any electronic means and whether or not transiently or incidentally to some other use of this publication) without written permission of the copyright holder except in accordance with the provisions of the Copyright, Designs and Patents Act 1988.

Applications for the copyright holder's written permission to reproduce any part of this publication should be addressed to the publishers.

This book is not endorsed by or affiliated with any website or organization mentioned in this book in any way.

Dedication:

To my Dad, Peter, who dedicated his life to helping others. May this book follow in your enormous footsteps.

You were a giant among men.

Acknowledgements

Thank you to everyone who has helped me on my journey to make this book a reality.

To my husband, John Chrisman for your steadfast support of my every endeavour, no matter how misguided or wacky. Thank you for supporting me 100%.

To all the doctors and researchers who paved the way to show that a whole plant foods lifestyle can help people prevent and even reverse lifestyle disease: Dr. Dean Ornish, Dr. Neal Barnard, Dr. Caldwell Esselstyn, Dr. T Collin Campbell, Dr. Nicholas Wright, Dr. John McDougall, Dr. Wendy Walrabenstein, Dr. Michael Greger and every health professional on earth who promotes a whole plant foods lifestyle for their patients.

Thank you.

Thank you to my beta readers: Dianne Doyle, Cheryl Eastwood, Tiffany Bokhari, Misty Young, Catherine Gordon, Celeste Mele, and Siiri Corby whose keen eyes and insights made this book better than I could have imagined.

Thank you to my friend and colleague Claire Williams for helping me stay focused and get past the finish line. (clairecreatescontent.com)

To my friend and mentor Wilene Dunne (wcdenterprises.com) for making the publishing journey less overwhelming.

To Mitali Deypurkaystha (theveganpublisher.com/) for providing me with a plan I could follow. I'd still be dreaming about writing a book without you.

To Peter Asprey (aspreycreative.com.au), the best cover designer in the world. Thank you so much for giving my message a face.

Thank you to YOU – for buying this book and having faith in me to guide you on your journey to Fabulous Health.

Praise for FABULOUS HEALTH

"Fabulous Health is a straightforward guide to changing your health and even saving your life. It is a treasury of solid health information, accompanied by practical tips to put that information to work for a broad range of health issues. I highly recommend it."

Neal D. Barnard, MD, FACC

Adjunct Associate Professor of Medicine, George Washington University School of Medicine

President, Physicians Committee for Responsible Medicine

"If you've ever wished for a compassionate, practical, and empowering guide to reclaim your health—look no further. Fabulous Health by Terri Chrisman is the real deal. With clarity, wisdom, and a whole lot of heart, Terri takes you by the hand and walks you through every step of transforming your life—starting with the food on your plate and reaching all the way to the thoughts in your head.

Terri's book is filled with actionable tools: how to stock your kitchen, what to eat, how to shop smart, and how to navigate real-world challenges without losing sight of your goals. She doesn't just help you eat better—she helps you live better.

What I love most is how approachable Fabulous Health is. Whether you're brand new to plant-based living or just need a refresh, Terri offers a judgment-free, science-backed roadmap to help you thrive.

This isn't just a book. It's a lifestyle manual, a cookbook, a pep talk, and a wake-up call all rolled into one.

I wholeheartedly recommend Fabulous Health to anyone ready to take control of their well-being and feel fabulous doing it!"

Chef AJ, Best-selling author of *Sweet Indulgence* and *The Secrets to Ultimate Weight Loss*

"Fabulous Health offers guidance and useful tips everyone can benefit from when they begin their plant based journey."

Jill McKeever. Plant-based YouTuber.

"Terri Chrisman's 'Fabulous Health' strikes a perfect balance between practical nutrition advice and thoughtful journal prompts. The reflection sections helped me examine my habits and behaviors in ways I never had before—they're not just supplementary but essential for creating lasting lifestyle changes. Packed with actionable tips, this book provides everything needed to transform your health journey and maintain wellness for the long term."

Dr Nitu Bajekal, Senior Consultant ObGyn and author of *Living PCOS Free* and *Finding Me in Menopause*

"A very thoughtful book for people who are looking to try a change and get their health back on track"

Dr. Nicholas Wright.
General Practitioner Fellow and author of The BROAD study

"If you're just getting started on a plant-based path and need more guidance than just recipes -- but those, too! -- then look no further. "Fabulous Health" is your partner, walking by your side, educating without preaching, so you can make informed decisions nutrition, forming good habits, and how to joyfully adopt this new lifestyle."

Miyoko Schinner, Bestselling Author, Founder and Board President of Rancho Compasión

Contents

Disclaimer 18
Introduction 19

CHAPTER 1: My Story 25
    Who Puts A Kid On A Diet At Age Four?
    Struggling With Weight
    Dead Dads Suck
    25 Years Later
    Why Am I Telling You All This?
        Workbook

CHAPTER 2: What Do You Want? 33
    Case Study: Wilene
    What Do You Want?
    Live For Now
        Workbook

CHAPTER 3: The Six Pillars of a Healthy Lifestyle 41
    Pillar 1—Plant-Based Nutrition
    Pillar 2—Physical Activity
    Pillar 3—Stress Reduction
    Pillar 4—Avoidance Of Smoking And Risky Behaviors
    Pillar 5—Restorative Sleep
    Pillar 6—Connection To Others
        Workbook

CHAPTER 4: What Diseases Can This Program Help? 47
    Cancer
    Diabetes
        Type 2 Diabetes
        Type 1 Diabetes
        Gestational Diabetes
        Alzheimer's Disease
    High Cholesterol (Dyslipidemia)
    Atherosclerosis

Heart Disease
High Blood Pressure (Hypertension)
  Exercise
  Salt
  Food and Blood Pressure
  Stress
Obesity
  Metabolic Syndrome
  Hormone Imbalances
Autoimmune Diseases
  Hashimotos
  Rheumatoid Arthritis
Reproduction Problems
  PCOS
Gut Issues
  Ulcerative Colitis and Crohn's Disease
  Irritable Bowel Syndrome
    Workbook

CHAPTER 5: The Broken System 71
The Bliss Point
The Obesogenic Environment
Food Deserts
Marketing
USDA Guidelines
Government Subsidies
  Workbook

CHAPTER 6: Nutrition 101 79
Macronutrients
  Alcohol
  Carbohydrates
  Protein
  Fat
Micronutrients
  Vitamins
  Minerals

- Phytonutrients
- Adaptogens
- Antinutrients
- Supplementation
  - Vitamin B12
  - Vitamin D
  - Calcium
  - Omega 3
  - Vitamin C
  - Multivitamins
    - Workbook

CHAPTER 7: A New Way of Eating 91
- What is ASOUPAS free?
  - Animal Products
  - Sugar
  - Oil
  - Ultra-Processed Foods
  - Alcohol
  - Salt
    - Workbook

CHAPTER 8: Setting Up For Success 99
- Know Your Numbers
  - Blood Tests
  - Body Measurements
  - Weight
  - Height
  - Anthropometric and Biometric Measurements
- Home Measurement Of Body Fat
  - Body Fat Calculation
- Other Measurements
- Starting Photos
- Goal Setting
  - Smart Goals
- It's Not All About Weight Loss
- Keep A Journal
- Tracking Progress
  - Workbook

CHAPTER 9: Changing Your Environment 113
    Clean Out The Junk
    Empty The Cabinets
    The Easy Drive-Through
    Living With Others
    Sodas And Sugar-Sweetened Beverages
    What About Sugar-Free Sodas?
        Workbook

CHAPTER 10: What's On The Menu? 119
    Nutrient Density Versus Energy Density
    What Foods Are On The Program?
    Why Are The Foods On The Left The Only Ones On The Program?
    Veggies
        Starchy Vegetables
        Non-starchy Vegetables
        Eat The Rainbow
    Whole Grains
    Fruit
        Fresh Or Frozen?
        Cans/Jars
    Beans And Legumes
    Herbs, Spices And Condiments
    Nuts And Seeds
    What About Coffee?
    Healthy Foods List
    Food Swaps
    Plant Protein
    Plant Calcium
    Plant-based B Vitamins
    Gluten-Free
        Workbook

CHAPTER 11: Let's Go Shopping 141
    Plan
    Write
    Eat
    Read
    The Ninja Strategy
        Workbook

CHAPTER 12: Food Labels 147
    Real Food Doesn't Need A Label
    Ingredients
    Deciphering The Food Label
        Workbook

CHAPTER 13: Kitchen Essentials 153
    Sharp Knives
    Vegetable Chopper
    High-Speed Blender
    Food Processor
    Instant Pot
    Pots And Pans
    Air Fryer
    Oven/Toaster Oven
    Microwave
        Workbook

CHAPTER 14: Organic Versus Conventional Produce 157
    Why Should You Eat Organic Food?
    Dirty Dozen
    Clean 15
        Workbook

CHAPTER 15: Transitional Foods 163
    Transitional Foods
    Vegan Versus Whole Plant Foods Diet
    Plant-Based Junk Food
        Fries
        Cupcakes
        Smoothie Bowls
    Plant-Based Meat Alternatives
    Plant-Based Cheese
        Nooch
    Cooking Without Oil
        Workbook

CHAPTER 16: Whole Plant Foods On A Budget 171
    Whole Plant Food Meals On A Budget
        Fruit and Vegetables

    Beans and Lentils
    Whole Grains
    Herbs
    Spices
    Buy In bulk
  Pantry Staples
  In The Freezer
    Workbook

CHAPTER 17: Be Prepared 179

Prepping
    Primary Prep—Once Per Week
    Secondary Prep—On The Fly
    Freeze It
Snacks
Prepped Frozen Meals
Meal Planning
    Workbook

CHAPTER 18: Nutrient Loading 185

Veggies For Breakfast
Eat Low Energy-density Foods First
Salad Prep Like A Boss!
    Workbook

CHAPTER 19: How to 'Plantify' Your Favorite Recipes 193

Swap it!
Basic Plantifying Formula
Spaghetti Bolognese
Tofu Guts
Cheese!
    Not Queso
    Tofu Ricotta
    Parmesan
Plant Milk
    Workbook

CHAPTER 20: Creating Healthy Habits 201

Make Habits Easy
Make Habits Replicable
Habit Stacking

Logging
Rewards For Behavior Change
    Workbook

CHAPTER 21: Putting It All Together 207
Three Easy Steps To Transitioning To A Whole Plant Foods Diet
    Step 1: Start With What You Already Like
    Step 2: Swap It Out
    Step 3: Try New Things
The 100% rule
Your Ex List
No Cheat Days
Progress Over Perfection
Every Bite Is Helping Or Hurting You
    Workbook

CHAPTER 22: Tackling Self-doubt 217
Have Faith
Be Kind To Yourself If You Slip Up
Measure More Than Scale Weight
Self Educate
    Workbook

CHAPTER 23: Life In The Real World 225
Travel
Eating At Restaurants
Parties
Family Holidays
Dealing with Negative People/Peer Pressure
Community
    Workbook

CHAPTER 24: Advanced Techniques 233
What To Do When You Plateau
The Ad Libitum Lie
The Sigh
Intermittent Fasting
Juicing Versus Smoothies
    Workbook

CHAPTER 25: What's Next? 241
    Yearly Checkups
    Reducing Medications
    Menopause
    Living Your Best Life
        Workbook

CHAPTER 26: Recipes 247
    Breakfast
        Veggies For Breakfast
        Granola
        Fruit Salad
        Soy Yogurt
        Scrambled Tofu
        Green Smoothie
        Purple Smoothie
        Pancakes
    Lunch And Dinner
        Basic Pasta Sauce
            Arrabiata
            Puttanesca
        Minestrone
        Bean Chili
        Risotto
        Shepherd's Pie
            DIY Parmesan
        Lasagne
            Cheesy Tofu Bechamel
        Black Bean and Tempeh Casserole
        Bean Burgers
        Mike's Butter Beans
    Extras
        Cheesy Sauce
            Mac'N'Cheeze
        Tofu Ricotta
        Tofu Mayo
        Mushroom Gravy
        Hummus
    Snacks
        Oat Cookies
        Tofu Chocolate Mousse
        Date Snickers

Chia And Banana Pudding
Gelato

Appendix 271
Quiz Answers

Bibliography 272
Resources 282
Index 284

Disclaimer

I am not a medical doctor. I am a university-qualified nutritionist with a master's degree in nutrition. I'm a board-certified diplomat of the American College of Lifestyle Medicine. This means I'm qualified to advise you on lifestyle modifications to improve your health. My advice is supported by scientific literature, and I provide references where appropriate. No self-help book should be a substitute for personal, individualized medical care. Please consult your primary care physician before undertaking this or any other lifestyle change. If you are on any medications, please monitor them carefully. As you become healthier, you may require less medication. NEVER alter or cease your medication without first consulting your primary care physician. They will adjust your medicines if and when it is appropriate for you.

This book considers lifestyle modifications to prevent non-communicable diseases but does not account for congenital genetic defects. If you suffer from a genetically based condition, the information in this book may help you maintain your health but cannot alleviate your condition.

This book is for information purposes only and does not replace medical advice of any form.

Introduction

Why You Need This Book

I lost my Dad to a massive heart attack when he was only fifty one years young. I've spent more of my life without my Dad than with him. I have a broken heart that will never mend. My Dad didn't know he had heart disease. He didn't know that the plaque in his arteries could kill him at any minute, and neither did I. If I could turn back time, I'd give my Dad this book. I'd help him see what lifestyle choices may have played a part in his untimely demise.

My Dad was unlucky. He didn't get a second chance. You have a second chance, and I'll see to it.

I've spent much of my adult life learning about the connection between lifestyle and noncommunicable diseases. (That's a scientific way of saying 'diseases we can't catch from other people').

Diseases like type 2 diabetes, coronary artery disease, high blood pressure, dementia, rheumatoid arthritis, cancer – and many others can be helped by lifestyle changes.

I'm convinced by the enormous mountain of scientific literature linking nutrition to health. In my private practice, I've helped people lose weight and reduce their risk of these debilitating diseases. I've even helped myself and my family. By following the practices I share in this book, I lowered my blood pressure, so I no longer need medication. I lost excess fat and know I'm doing my best for my body.

Adopting a healthy lifestyle is not just for me. It's for you, too. Search the internet for whole plant foods diet success stories, and you'll find thousands of people who have improved their health, reduced medications, and sometimes reversed disease by changing what they eat.

I hope this book speaks to you and awakens a desire to be the captain of your ship. To steer your life away from disease and toward health so that you can partner with your health professionals and take positive steps towards health and vitality. Please don't be a passive passenger. Take control and choose your own destiny.

Who This Book Is For

- This book is for people who want to live their lives at a healthy weight, free of worry about lifestyle diseases.
- This book is for people who have tried everything, and yet they still are at risk of ill health or continue to carry the burden of disease.
- This book is for people who do not want to spend their lives weighing and measuring their food.
- This book is for people who are sick of yo-yo dieting.
- This book is for people who are sick and tired of being sick and tired.
- This book is for people who hate cooking and also for people who want to be gourmet chefs.
- This book is for people already diagnosed with lifestyle-based conditions such as high blood pressure, high cholesterol, diabetes, pre-diabetes, fatty liver, metabolic syndrome, PCOS, IBS, Crohn's disease, ulcerative colitis, rheumatoid arthritis or any manner of immune system conditions.
- This book is for people who want to be healthy without the disabling symptoms of lifestyle disease or the debilitating side effects of the drugs used to manage them.

Who This Book Is NOT For

- This book is not for you if you are recovering from or currently have an eating disorder. Please seek assistance from your primary physician and access resources specific to your situation.
- This book is not intended for children. Children have specific nutrient requirements to ensure optimal nutrition whilst growing. If you believe your child could benefit from nutrition counseling, please contact me privately or consult your doctor.
- If you are trying to gain weight, use this book as a guide. However, you will need to add more high-calorie plant foods. Please contact me personally, and I can formulate a weight gain plan for you using whole plant foods.
- This is not a diet book. If you want to lose 20 pounds this weekend, then go back to eating your usual unhealthy diet, this is not the book for you.
- This book is not for you if you think reading it will change your life. You must take action steps to change your health. Just reading won't cut it. There is "doing" to be done. I promise that if you follow the program described in this book to the letter, you will reap the rewards of better health.

What You Can Expect

From the outset, you need to know that this book promotes a whole plant foods lifestyle. That means that I will ask you to stop eating animal products in all forms. If this scares you, don't worry; I have your back. I will help you make the transition to a whole plant foods lifestyle as easy and delicious as possible. I have collated many easy tasty recipes that mimic your favorite animal-based foods without excess fat, cholesterol, and other unhealthy ingredients.

Don't stress. I understand that we are all on our own journey of health discovery. It might take you some time to remove unhealthy foods from your life altogether, and you might fall off the wagon a couple of times, but eventually you will start feeling so fabulous that those unhealthy foods will have no power over you. Having said that, if you want true transformation in a minimal amount of time, follow the program from the outset – cold turkey (please forgive the pun) – and you will reap the most significant benefit.

You can be sure that all the information contained in this book is backed by solid scientific evidence. I have provided references where appropriate. In the resources section, I have linked to a few of my favorite doctors, non-governmental organizations, and other leaders in the field of health to provide additional evidence.

Lastly, expect to have your mind blown! Expect to learn facts about the food industry that you did not think were ethical or even possible. Expect to be awakened to the realization that no one cares about your health but you, and that you have the power to make lasting positive change in your health.

I have faith in you. **YOU CAN DO IT!**

The Book Structure

This book is part information, part practical steps to implement, and part practical workbook. At the end of each chapter are questions to answer and space for you to journal your thoughts. Please don't skip these pages. They are vital. I can't tell you how many books I have read only to forget the details soon after.

By doing short, easy quizzes and taking notes, you are more likely to retain the information. Plus, your notes will be in YOUR words, so they will resonate with you and help you on YOUR journey.

Promise me now that you will use these sections to your best advantage. You can thank me later.

FAQ

Have you got questions? I've got answers.

Will it work for me?

If you have been habitually eating the Standard American Diet (SAD) of fast food, meat, dairy, and processed foods, you will see amazing results when you start following my guidance. It's up to you how much you want to follow the advice. In the scientific community we call this a 'dose-response'. This means that the more closely you follow the advice in this book, the better results you will get.

Do I have to follow a meal plan?

The short answer is no. However, I recognize that everyone's journey is different, and I have provided some suggested plans if you prefer to follow a plan. I have made this program so easy that you can create your own plan that suits your lifestyle by following simple guidelines.

Will I be hungry?

Absolutely not! You can eat as much as you like until you are fully satisfied. Want some more chips? Go ahead and have some. The caveat here is 'fully satisfied'. As you will learn in this book, calories are important. Eating every meal until you are bursting at the seams will not help you on your health journey. Don't worry, I promise you won't go hungry. Ever.

How much effort will it take?

Like all things, it takes time to get into new habits. Initially, it might seem a little daunting, but I promise that fully immersing yourself in this way of life will become easy very quickly. And the payoff will be so huge that you will never want to return to your old way of eating again.

Am I going to have to give up my favorite foods?

If your favorite foods are donuts, fast-food hamburgers, and soft drinks, then yes. I will introduce you to a whole new world of deliciously tantalizing new foods that are so tasty and satisfying, those unhealthy options will no longer interest you. I will also offer you new ways to prepare your favorite recipes that make them healthier and just as delicious as the ones you have grown to love.

Are there cheat days built in?

No, there are not. You are the captain of your own destiny. You choose how healthy you want to be. The more you stray from a healthy lifestyle, the less effective it will be. Will that mean you can't have cake on your birthday? Not at all. Have the cake. Just make it a healthy cake and eat it with no guilt.

If you accidentally fall off the wagon – no worries – just brush yourself off and get back on the program. We are all human. Over time, these lapses will become less and less frequent as the old way of eating will no longer appeal to you.

Do I need specialized equipment?

It is not imperative, but I highly recommend some specialized kitchen appliances. Having the right equipment makes everything so much easier. If you do not have these appliances, you can certainly use the kitchen equipment you already have. Purchase the absolute best appliances you can afford. You can always scour thrift stores or eBay for second-hand ones, keep an eye on department store sales, or hint to loved ones at gift-giving times.

The equipment I use daily is included in Chapter 13.

How To Use This Book

1. Read everything. Don't skim read, fully read. Reread it if you don't completely understand the concepts.

2. Do the quizzes and answer the questions at the end of each chapter. Even if you think you understand the topic. If you believe the question doesn't relate to you – or you think you have nothing to say, give it a go anyway. Try to fill out everything you can.

3. Please don't try to do this alone. Talk about it. Discuss what you are learning with your friends and family. They may not instantly support you on your journey, but having at least one person in your corner for when times get tough is essential. I cannot stress enough how important community is when you are making changes such as the ones in this book.

4. Fill in the journal. At the end of every chapter is a space for journaling. This is where you write your thoughts, affirmations and emotions. This is a space for you to connect with the material fully and how it is relevant to you. Please don't ignore this part. It's more potent than you might think.

This is your safe space. Anything you add to your journal is entirely private. I cannot see what you write in your journal nor anyone else. So, use this to express yourself.

Research shows that the more you are exposed to a new idea, the better your chance of understanding it. We all learn in different ways. For some, it will click just by reading, and for people like me – I'm a kinesthetic learner—I love to do the work myself. That's why I have incorporated quizzes in every module.

By the time you have finished this book, I expect it to have dog-eared pages, sticky notes highlighted sections and scribbles in the margins. This is your book. This is your life. How you learn is up to you. Please don't just read this book and put it back on the shelf out of sight out of mind. Put yourself into this program so you can reap the rewards.

5. Join the online community. I've created an exclusive Facebook group for those who have purchased the book. Here, you can share your wins and challenges or just hang out with cool people on the same journey. Head over to fabuloushealthbook.net/bonuses and join the community.

6. Pick up some sweet bonuses. In appreciation of your buying this book – for which I am eternally grateful, I've put together a bunch of sweet bonuses that will help you on your journey. I update them constantly, so head over to fabuloushealthbook.net/bonuses to get your freebies.

**Are you ready to live a life of Fabulous Health?
Come with me and let's get cracking!**

CHAPTER 1: My Story

What's In This Chapter?

It is vital that you get to know me as you read this book. You need to know that I have struggled with my weight, and, like you, I'm concerned about my long-term health. I have searched for answers and solutions to improve my health and fitness for my entire life. When I finally found methods that work and that are based on science, I wanted to share my learning and experiences with you. I hope my journey resonates and my teaching enriches your life. My health and your health are my top priorities.

Who Puts A Kid On A Diet At Age Four?

I was a fat kid. I was put on a diet at the age of four by my doctor. Of course, I don't remember that, but I remember being 'chunky' during my childhood.

My Dad was fat, and all his sisters were obese. I just figured that we came from a fat family. I watched them struggle every day, trying every diet or pill available, weighing all their food, but nothing ever worked for them. No matter what they did, they were always obese.

My Mum, on the other hand, is trim and has never struggled with her weight. If anything, she has to work to keep herself from getting too thin. She is in her eighties now and is as fit as a fiddle. She's the same size she was when she was married. She goes hiking weekly, participates in bushwalking club and calisthenics club, walks to the supermarket, and travels around the countryside towing her caravan (RV) behind her. She is an action woman! I sincerely believe she is so fit and sprightly because of her diet. She eats mainly healthy fruit, veggies, whole grains, minimal animal products, and very little processed food. She never gets takeout or eats candy and rarely goes to a restaurant.

When we were kids, Mum always made sure we ate healthy food. She shopped at the farmers market twice weekly to stock up on fresh fruit and veggies. When I was growing up, there were rarely any sodas, sweets, or snack foods in our house. Our dessert options were either fruit or vanilla ice cream. As I didn't like ice cream, my option was fruit.

We always had lots of fresh, healthy food in our home, but I was more like my Dad when it came to eating. While Mum treated food as fuel necessary for survival, Dad and I LOVED food. We loved the texture, the taste, and the pleasure of food. You couldn't bring donuts into our house without Dad and me scoffing most of them.

It wasn't the food my Mum fed me that made me gain weight; it was the snacks I sneaked between meals.

Next door to my elementary school was a fish and chip shop. After school, I would save my fifty-cent allowance and buy twenty-cents of chips and four potato cakes. That's about 3000 calories of deep-fried potatoes and batter. It was heaven, but it wasn't great for my health.

As I matured, I fought with my flab by enrolling in lots of sports. The exercise helped me to keep my weight down and allowed me to eat the foods I loved. It worked, too, but as I grew older, keeping thin became more challenging than ever.

At sixteen, my parents took me to a dietitian who put me on a restricted-calorie diet that only made me hungry and grumpy. She made me eat tinned fruit and wheat germ for breakfast. It was like eating cardboard – absolutely hideous. I learned right then that restrictive diets where you are made to eat food you don't like are not sustainable.

Struggling With Weight

When I was eighteen and getting chunkier by the day, I became vegetarian. I had this ridiculous notion that I could lose weight by giving up a major food group. I was not a great fan of meat, but I was a fan of chocolate, so the meat went, and the chocolate stayed. Back then, my logic was not based on science.

Later, I learned more about factory farming and the torture animals endured. I learned being vegetarian was beneficial not only to my health but also to the planet's health. My logic was rudimentary and flawed but altruistic nonetheless.

After I left home, without the guidance of my healthy Mum, I was not as health-conscious as I should have been. I could buy a croissant or a cupcake any time I wanted, and Mum was not there to stop me. After all, cupcakes and croissants are vegetarian. As are cheese, fries, potato chips, and alcohol!

By age twenty-one, I was at my heaviest—80 kg—almost 180 pounds! I had no clue what I was doing. I was drinking a lot of alcohol and going out partying all the time – late-night snacking was normal. I just figured that, like my Dad and his sisters, I was 'heavy set.'

Over the years, I managed to lose weight, but I put it on again multiple times. I just couldn't seem to stay trim. I tried many diets, none of which worked very well because I had no plan. I would try to give up chocolate, wine, potatoes, or something else without knowing what I was doing. My weight bounced around like a yo-yo. Sometimes, I was happy with my weight, and other times, not so much. Looking back on these struggles, I now realize I was looking to lose weight for the wrong reasons. I was more concerned with fitting into skinny jeans than keeping my arteries clean.

I joined a program where I ate only pre-packaged diet food. It was expensive and processed, and after a while, it became boring and monotonous. I did lose a lot of weight eating this way, but it was very restrictive, and I always felt I was denying myself the foods I wanted.

As soon as I started cooking for myself, the weight went back on. Not all at once, but slowly, it all came back over time.

I got very skinny following a self-imposed restrictive eating regimen. After my kids were born, I virtually starved myself to stay thin. My husband jokes that I lived on rocket (arugula) salad and champagne. It was no joke. To stay thin, I ate lettuce and ran five miles daily. Who can do that forever? Not me!

I tried calorie counting, weighing everything I ate, and macro counting.

These methods also worked well as long as I wrote everything down and weighed everything. Believe it or not, I did this for years, logging every morsel of food. Let me tell you, logging everything you eat is not the way to mental stability and food freedom! I still have the little notebooks full of calorie and macro calculations, reminding me of the food and diet dungeon I had created.

When I read these notebooks now, it seems evident that I had an eating disorder. At the time, I did not think so. I thought I was disciplined and following a plan – no matter how crazy that plan was. Nothing was sustainable for long because sooner or later, I'd cave in and have peanut butter on toast, leading to cupcakes, fries, and margaritas!

During all this time—about twenty years—I was slowly educating myself about nutrition. I was trying everything I could to biohack my body—the body I was born with, with the 'fat genes' (remember them?) to maintain a slim physique. All this research led me to understand that the way to health was through whole plant foods, not starvation diets. I loved veggies and continued to eat what I thought was the healthiest vegetarian diet—but I still struggled to keep at my goal weight. I didn't know that some of the foods I thought were healthy were not. It can be frustrating to think you are doing all the right things, but the scale just doesn't move.

I was vegetarian for over twenty-five years except for a short period of time when I ate chicken breast because I thought I needed more protein (spoiler alert—I did not need more protein). I finally decided to become vegan in 2015. I had been reading the scientific literature about the health consequences and environmental impact of animal products, especially dairy products. I decided that I could no longer contribute to animal suffering and the planet's devastation caused by animal agriculture. So, I ditched the dairy and eggs for good.

If you are unfamiliar with the vegan diet, it involves avoiding all animal products. That means no meat, poultry, eggs, cheese, milk, fish or seafood, gelatin (gummy bears), or honey. Veganism also has moral and ethical implications, which I will explain more about in Chapter 15.

Dead Dads Suck

Let's head back a bit so you can understand why I was on this perpetual diet rollercoaster.

When I was twenty-five, my entire world was shattered when my Dad, who was my favorite person in the whole world, died suddenly and unexpectedly at the tender age of fifty-one. He died younger than I am now. He had what doctors call a 'widowmaker' heart attack, a complete blockage of the arteries that supply the blood to the heart. He died instantly. He never even knew he had heart disease. He thought he was fit and healthy.

I'll never forget my Mum's words. When she told me, she didn't say that he died; she said he was killed. It's true. He didn't just die; he was killed, senselessly, unnecessarily, and pointlessly. It was like his own body murdered him. It was a devastating blow to my family, and I still miss him more than 30 years later. Even though it was a surprise to us, that heart attack did not come 'out of the blue'. His early and untimely death was the result of years of being overweight and years of eating animal products, fried food, and saturated fat.

My Dad was overweight his entire life. We ate healthy food at home, but that was another story altogether when he was out. He would have six dim sims (deep-fried meat parcels wrapped in pastry) for morning tea! His best friend owned a company called Mr.Donut, and you can guess that Dad regularly visited this friend and his yummy business. As a child, I hoped my arms would grow long enough so that when I hugged him, my fingers could wrap around his body and touch each other. That never happened, not even when I was an adult.

Dad knew he needed to look after his health, but he had no idea how to change his eating habits. He tried every diet under the sun, but he had no idea what he ate was killing him. In the 1970s and 1980s, his doctor prescribed diet pills, which were no more than what we call *speed* today. I vowed not to end up like my Dad or his surviving sisters. They were morbidly obese and perpetually on the diet roller coaster, endlessly searching for the magic pill, the magic food that would make them thin.

25 Years Later . . .

In 2015, I returned to university for a master's degree in nutrition, believing that I would be thin and healthy forever once I had all the knowledge. Even at university, I wasn't taught how to be healthy and avoid being fat. Three years of study and tens of thousands of dollars later, I still felt like something was missing. I was reading the latest science, yet the university system was still stuck in the dark ages.

One of my university assignments was to prescribe a high-calcium diet to an elderly patient with low calcium levels. The latest scientific literature pointed toward plant-based foods and away from dairy foods. So, I wrote the paper thinking I was at the cutting edge of scientific discovery – only to receive a C-grade from my professor for "having an agenda". Of course I had an agenda! An agenda to speak the truth. An agenda to present the latest scientific research and spread the word that dairy foods are not healthy for the human body. Well, that backfired.

I called upon a plant-based colleague in one of my university classes. She said, "Terri, give them what they want so you get the degree, then go into the world and spread the truth". That hit me hard. Didn't the university want to know the truth? Didn't they want to teach the truth?

It alerted me to the politics of education and the need to find the truth for ourselves. Even today, as I write this book years later, both USDA and Australian food guidelines promote the daily intake of dairy foods, which are known to promote cancer [1, 2].

At university, instead of learning what foods to eat to be the healthiest, I learned about the chemistry of nutrients in the human body and all the vitamins and minerals. This was important, but it didn't address the problem I was personally facing. I learned about the diseases of starvation and how to avoid obesity on a population level. Still, I didn't learn the secret to sustainable health until later.

When I finally found what works, I immersed myself in the literature again. In 2022, after another year of intense scientific study, I became board certified by the American College of Lifestyle Medicine. This is when it all came together—knowing there is a proven way to stay trim and healthy. A revelation was that most common diseases can be avoided or treated with food and lifestyle. I finally found what I was looking for, and I will share it with you.

Why Am I Telling You All This?

I am on a mission to help as many people as possible to lead happy and healthy lives. Not just fit into nice clothes. Perhaps my story resonates with you. Maybe you are doing everything right, but nothing seems to work. I want to help you get off that diet rollercoaster and be healthy now and forever. I want you to avoid the pain associated with being overweight and obese. I want you to stop spending money on medications and spend that money on yourself. I want you to stop spending time with your doctor and, instead, spend that time with those you love.

I want you to have real, lasting health free of disease. I'm talking about feeling good in your own skin. Feeling confident and attractive. I want you to be able to climb a mountain or jog without pain. Or play with your kids and grandkids without getting puffed. I want you to say 'yes' to the stairs instead of the elevator. I also don't want anyone to go through the trauma and heartache that I went through after losing my Dad. I don't want anyone to feel the tremendous pain that I felt (and still feel to this day), the pain of losing someone. I don't want you to lose your dad, your mum, your sister, or worse, your own life.

Being fat is not just uncomfortable and unsightly; it's a danger to your health. Being overweight or obese is a risk factor for a myriad of lifestyle diseases, including heart disease, stroke, Alzheimer's, diabetes, and even cancer.

What I just shared is crucial because I care about your health as much as I care about my health. Illness and death from obesity-related diseases can be avoidable if you have the correct information and eat the right foods.

I spent twenty years searching for the best lifestyle for my body, and I am absolutely convinced that it will work for you too. This is a lifestyle that is sustainable for the long term. The food is delicious and enjoyable, nourishing you without feeling deprived or as though you're missing out on flavor. This is not some fad diet promising you will lose 10 pounds in a weekend. This is a lifestyle backed by science. I know that I want only the best scientific information when I make decisions about my health, and I'm sure you feel the same way.

With my educational background and expertise, you can trust that the health advice I provide is grounded in science. This advice will guide you toward achieving a long, healthy, and fulfilling life. I hold a master's degree in nutrition, which gives me a solid understanding of the science behind nutrition. However, I want to emphasize that I didn't create this knowledge; I'm simply following the insights of the world's leading experts and sharing that information with you. The approach to eating that I'm about to teach you is based on years of scientific research. I'll introduce you to these experts and their research throughout the book.

Have you ever heard the quote attributed to the ancient Greek physician Hippocrates? He said, "Let food be thy medicine, and medicine be thy food".

Although today's modern doctors are taught virtually nothing of nutrition in their years at medical school (the sad truth), this old Greek dude pretty much hit the nail on the head.

OK – are you ready? I want to hear you shout it.

YES! I'M READY. BRING IT ON!!!!

Workbook

Quiz

There is no quiz for Chapter 1

Journal

Think about what's been holding you back in the past. What stories are you telling yourself that prevent you from making lasting change.

_____

_____

_____

_____

_____

_____

_____

_____

_____

_____

Quick Tip

The road to fabulous health is a lifelong journey. For some, results may come quickly, while for others, they may take time and persistence. Stay the course, trust the process, and I promise the results will come.

CHAPTER 2: What Do You Want?

"Whether you think you can or you think you can't, you are always right."
Henry Ford

What's In This Chapter?

In this chapter, we will define precisely what you want from life and health. You will need to consider what is important to you and why you want to improve your health. First, I will share an empowering story about a client.

Case Study: Wilene

I have a good friend, Wilene. She is the most amazing woman. She is an entrepreneur, a dog mum to five gorgeous pups, and the most generous soul who hosts lunches for friends and family every week. And she understands the power of how words can shape our lives. She is a business coach who helps people use words to create the life of their dreams. I'm all for that because I'm a very positive person. If I think it, I believe it, and I do it.

When I first met Wilene, she weighed 245 pounds. She was uncomfortable in her own body. She had pain, and she was using food as a drug. When she ate certain foods, they made her sleepy, which gave her an excuse not to do what was on her to-do list. When we met, she was sleeping so much in the daytime that it adversely affected her business.

After working with me for a couple of weeks, Wilene no longer took naps during the day, and the pain in her neck and shoulders disappeared. She was getting her work done, and she was thriving. Over a few months, she lost over forty pounds, and as I write this, Wilene is still losing weight. By changing her diet and being more thoughtful about fueling her body with quality food, she immediately began to feel better.

I was so impressed by her progress that I asked her to tell me what made her so successful. She told me that she decided to be healthy and used her words to make that health a reality in her life. She chose to live a healthier life—not a life by default but a life by design. She knew what she wanted, and she went for it—100%. And guess what? She got exactly what she wanted.

To watch the podcast with Wilene, watch episode 52 of The Fabulous Health Show Podcast (fabuloushealth.net/fabulous-health-show).

What Do You Want?

Do you want to be free of pain? Do you want to fit into your college clothes? Do you want to reverse your lifestyle illness so you don't have to take medication anymore? Do you want to make sure you are around to enjoy your grandchildren? Whatever you want, you need to know what it is, and you need to own it. Even if you think it is impossible. Even if you think you can't do it. I want to stop you right now and share my favorite quote. It's from Henry Ford.

"Whether you think you CAN or you think you CAN'T, you are always RIGHT".

Stop thinking that you can't, and start thinking that you CAN. Directly after that, start saying that you WILL. If you tell yourself you will be healthy, I will do my best to help you get there. I know you can do it. I will be here every step of the way. Just have faith in the process, take the required actions, and your life will change in ways you cannot even imagine right now.

Maybe you've never pictured yourself thin or have been sick so long that you can't imagine being healthy. Before you give up, stop. Forget the finish line—there isn't one. This is about living a long, healthy, happy life, and I can help you change how you live it.

Live For Now

All I want you to think about is now. What are you doing now? How are you feeling now? What choices are you making now? If you dwell on the past ("I used to be an athlete, now I get puffed walking up the stairs") or the future ("I'll never have six-pack abs"), all you are doing is adding stress and doubt. Leave that stuff behind! It does not, and will not, ever serve you well. Take a moment to be selfish. Not at the expense of others, of course, but by putting your health first and foremost in every situation. It doesn't mean that you should be self-absorbed and blind to others' needs, but it does mean that you prioritize your health in every situation.

For example, you're going to a football game and know that all the food options will be unhealthy. You plan to either eat at home beforehand or bring healthy snacks. You still enjoy the game with your friends and family without compromising your health goals. How easy was that?

In the sixth century BC, Chinese philosopher Lau Tzu reportedly said, *"The journey of 1000 miles begins with just one step."*

You are at the beginning of your thousand miles. Just take a deep breath and relax. Pretend it's not a thousand miles but only one mile. Or half a mile or just a few steps. You can do that, can't you? Of course you can!

When looking to improve our health, one of the first things people focus on is weight loss. However, I will ask you now not to focus on weight loss. Don't get me wrong, the weight loss will happen. Instead, focus on your daily actions. Each daily action will lead to weight loss and better health. Weight loss is the result of your daily actions. So, only weigh yourself once per week. If the scale is not your friend on any given day, and you know that you have been following all your daily action steps, give yourself a pat on the back and forget about it. The scale is just one data point. That rusty ol' piece of junk has no control over you. Move on.

However, the scale can also reflect your failure to do your daily actions. Be honest with yourself. Have you been inconsistent with daily healthy habits? Then you need to step up your game. This program works. However, it will not work if you choose not to do it. It's not a magic pill. There is work to be done and effort needed.

So, how do you get from where you are now to where you want to be? First, acknowledge where you are. Make no excuses for how you got here. Blame no person, no circumstance, no situation. You are where you are, and that is it. OWN IT!

Then, look forward. What will your life look like in three months, six months, five years? Imagine how fabulous you will feel when you are healthy and free from the struggle of excess weight and illness. It may seem hard now, but do your best to try. You can do it, so let your imagination run wild.

Close your eyes. See yourself a year from now, five years from now, living your best life. What do you look like? Are you slim and healthy? Who is with you? What are you doing?

Are you lying on a beach soaking up the sun, confident in your own body? Are you effortlessly trekking up a mountain to see the sunset, feeling your strong, fit legs carry you forward? Are you chasing your kids around the park, laughing instead of wheezing and out of breath? Are you slinking into a teeny tiny airline seat and heading off on an adventure of a lifetime?

Imagine feeling fit, healthy, disease-free, and able to do everything you want. You are confident in your skin, you feel sexy and attractive in your clothes, you are proud of your fitness, and you enjoy life to the fullest.

Just bask in this image for a few moments. Really feel it. Don't be fearful of it. Embrace it. At this point, there may be tears. I know because I have shed them myself. It's okay to feel miserable about your present circumstance, but only for an instant. Because right now, you will say goodbye to that unhealthy version of yourself and hello to a newer, healthier, happier version. You may be at rock bottom today, and the only way is up! You do not have to do this on your own. I've got your back.

I understand how scary change can be. It can be daunting and overwhelming. Don't stress on that. Take it one step at a time. Don't worry about the details. Stick with me and have faith that everything is going to be alright. You have entrusted me to look after you, and I will. Don't think about how hard it's going to be. Think about how much fun we will have together. Think about how fabulous you will feel. That's what it's all about.

Each chapter in this book has a journaling space to reflect on what you have learned and how to incorporate that knowledge into your life. There will be reflection exercises, action steps, and maybe some homework.

Please don't skip past these steps. This is the most crucial part of your journey. Use this book as a tool. If this book doesn't look like it's been through the washing machine twenty times by the time you have finished it, you are not using it properly. I want you to highlight, post sticky notes, doodle, journal your feelings, and anything else you need to do to help you on your journey.

For today's exercise, have a frank conversation with yourself. Why are you here, and what do you want? Then please take time to fill in your journal. Feel free to add any additional thoughts.

> **Quick Tip**
>
> Rather than considering this program as a diet, consider it your lifestyle going forward. If you want ultimate success and freedom from weight gain and ill health, adopt this as your new normal. Don't stress about this; you will build on habits, one at a time. Take it easy and enjoy the process.

Workbook

What do I want? (Answer these questions)

Precisely, what do I want for my life?

_____
_____
_____

What am I doing right now that will help me get what I want?

_____
_____
_____

What am I doing right now that is hindering me from getting what I want?

_____
_____
_____
_____

What will my life look like in five years once I am healthy? (Dream BIG and describe it in detail).

_____
_____
_____

Additional thoughts.

_____
_____
_____
_____
_____

NOTES:

CHAPTER 3: The Six Pillars Of A Healthy Lifestyle

"The answer to the American health crisis is the food that each of us chooses to put in our mouths each day. It's as simple as that." T. Colin Campbell, PhD

What's In This Chapter?

In this chapter, I will discuss the six pillars of a healthy life, which I learned at the American College of Lifestyle Medicine. If you nail these, you will be on your way to a life of health and vitality.

Pillar 1 — Plant-Based Nutrition

Plants are the key to lasting health and optimal nutrition. There are many scientific studies and reports on the dangers of saturated fat, cholesterol, processed meat, and ultra-processed foods. All the science on whole plant foods points to how awesome they are to your health. Even health organizations and governments are finally getting on board. The Canadian dietary guidelines ditched dairy products as a food group [3]. The German guidelines recommend eating 75% plant foods [4]. As I write this book, Australians and Americans are updating their guidelines. I'm putting my money on them both, promoting more plant food for health. I will spend most of this book on plant-based nutrition, but there are other things you can do to keep yourself healthy.

Pillar 2 — Physical Activity

Exercise is awesome! We are human beings with bones, muscles, and joints that are made to run, jump, bend, and get sweaty. The human body was not designed to sit in a chair all day. It was designed to move.

Exercise is the best drug on the planet with hardly any side effects – except for feeling fantastic!

Exercise works as effectively as medication to prevent disease.

In a trial of 3234 patients with pre-diabetes, participants were prescribed either a diabetes medication (metformin) or an exercise program. They were followed for 2.8 years to see if either treatment reduced the risk of developing diabetes. The people who exercised were half as likely to develop diabetes than those who took the medication [5].

Exercise can also lower blood pressure. During exercise, blood pressure rises due to the increased need for the heart to pump faster and send more blood to the muscles. After exercise, blood pressure reduces and stays low. The fitter you become, the lower your blood pressure becomes. Exercise can be as effective at lowering blood pressure as low-dose medication [6].

Exercise is also an effective treatment against depression [7]. Again, researchers found that exercise was just as effective as medications and therapy. Even better results occurred when exercise was combined with medication and therapy. Any exercise works. Walking, jogging, dancing, yoga, and strength training were all beneficial. Find what gives you joy, and go ahead and do it.

Most countries recommend 150 minutes of moderate or 75 minutes of vigorous exercise per week. This equates to 30 minutes of sprightly walking, whereby you can talk but not sing, five times per week. How about three 25-minute pickleball games? Or jump around to your favorite tunes in your living room for 20 minutes daily. You can do that, right? So, get out there and MOVE!

Pillar 3 — Stress Reduction

Stress is the pandemic of the 21st century. It seems everyone is under stress. Financial stress, family stress, and work stress. It's killing you – literally. Have you heard of the 'fight or flight' mechanism? This is part of your sympathetic nervous system. It sets your body up for conflict. It helps you get back on the sidewalk when you accidentally step in front of a bus. It enables you to survive.

What if you are just hanging out at home, worrying? Or your boss gave you a hard deadline you know you can't meet? Or you forgot your partner's birthday? All this is stressful. And it's unhealthy.

Acute stress can save your life (get back on that curb!), but chronic stress can shorten it. The stress response sets off a cascade of hormones, including cortisol. Cortisol makes you hungry, and it stores fat [8]. Under stress, adrenaline peaks. When you have excess adrenaline at times when it's not needed, your heart rate increases, which puts you at risk of high blood pressure and strokes.

Reducing stress can be as simple as moving away from the stressor (your boss?) and taking a few minutes to collect your thoughts. Deep abdominal breathing can lower the stress response within minutes.

If you cannot remove the stress, find a way to combat it by distancing yourself from it. For example, if you have financial stress, think of ways to save money. Set up a savings plan. Seek financial advice and formulate a solution. It might not solve all your financial issues, but you will be doing your best to fix the problem and reduce your stress. For action steps to help reduce stress, head to Chapter 4.

Pillar 4—Avoidance Of Smoking And Risky Behaviors

We all know that smoking is not good for us, right? Smoking is responsible for 90% of lung cancer deaths [9]. Smoking also raises blood pressure [10]. Yet, some people still smoke. You know it's not healthy. So, the next time you think about lighting up, consider all the work you do for your health. Does smoking support your goals? Does it align with the person you want to be?

What about alcohol? Drinking is entwined with our culture. It's what we do when we celebrate. Sometimes, it's part of our identity. Is that the identity you want? Does drinking help you lose weight? Does it align with the person you want to be? Find out why its a good idea to remove alcohol from your life in Chapter 7.

Substance addiction is personal and complex. This book does not address addiction to anything other than food. If you use drugs, alcohol, or tobacco, consider reaching out for help from service providers that are trained in substance abuse. See the resources sections as a starting place to get help to quit.

Pillar 5—Restorative Sleep

Never underestimate sleep. Sleep is so vital to our health. When we sleep, our bodies are busy repairing tissue, making memories, and regulating hormones. Most of us are oblivious to so much going on in the night shift. When you don't give your body enough sleep, all that repair work only gets half done, and you feel the effects the next day. If this is a regular occurrence, you can compromise your health. People who suffer from short-duration and disrupted sleep patterns are two times more at risk of developing obesity than people with optimal sleep patterns [11]. In addition, sub-optimal sleep can increase your risk for diabetes, high cholesterol, high blood pressure, and heart attacks.

Here are some ways to improve your sleep duration and quality. Try them out and see what works for you.

- Go to bed and get out of bed at the same time every day, weekdays and weekends. Aim to have between seven and nine hours of quality sleep each night. Start when you need to wake up and work backward to find your bedtime.
- Have a bedtime routine. This is called sleep hygiene. Set an alarm on your device 30—60 minutes before sleep time and start getting ready

for bed. Put on your jammies, brush your teeth, and turn the lights down. This will set your mind up for sleep, and you will start getting tired.

- Turn off those dang devices! Computerized devices with screens emit blue light that keeps your neurons firing and your brain awake. No computers, TVs, or cell phones at least 90 minutes before bed.
- If you are not tired, try reading. Not on the iPad, a real paper book. Hey! I have an idea. How about you read this book before bed each night? Reading will tire your brain out. (hopefully, not because the book is boring!)
- Don't drink alcohol or eat sugar before bed.
- Eat an early dinner and have most of your starchy carbohydrates earlier in the day.
- If you can't fall asleep because you exercise after dinner, switch your exercise to earlier in the day.
- Ensure your room is dark and cool.

Pillar 6 — Connection To Others

Being part of a community — whether a social circle, a community group, or friends with people who share common interests — benefits your health. Humans thrive when we can share our experiences with others. Connecting with others we care about helps lower stress and activates the parasympathetic nervous system (part of our central nervous system that promotes rest and recovery).

A Harvard University study following 456 men for 75 years found that connectedness with others was the most important predictor of happiness and longevity [12]. The study found that close relationships, more than money or fame were what kept people happy and that these relationships helped delay mental and physical decline more so than social class, IQ or genetics.

Being socially isolated is a risk factor for dementia, including Alzheimer's disease. The 2020 Lancet Report on Dementia Prevention Intervention and Care lists social isolation as one of the 12 risk factors for developing dementia [13]. It also states that having healthy social relationships throughout life can slow down cognitive decline and protect against damage to the aging brain.

If you feel lonely and you are alone for more of your day than not, I urge you to reach out and find your tribe. Making new friends can be daunting and scary. You can search online for groups of people in your area who share the same interests. Do you like knitting? Find your local knitting circle. Do you like playing sports? Join a local sporting club.

If you can't leave your home, there are places online to find your people. It doesn't matter if you are shy; just turn up, log in, and watch.

Soon enough, you will discover if you have chosen the right group. If not, move on and try again. I know that your people are out there somewhere for you. You just have to find them.

Workbook

Quiz

Answer True or False.

1. A healthy lifestyle includes six pillars: plant-based nutrition, absence of risky behaviors, meaningful connection to others, restorative sleep, stress reduction, and adequate physical activity.

2. Phones and tablets emit blue light that can keep my brain awake and make sleeping difficult.

3. Moderate red wine drinking is okay as it contains polyphenols that are good for health.

4. If I exercise according to the guidelines, I can stop all my medications.

ANSWERS in Appendix

Journal

Today I learned
_____

Today I feel
_____

I am proud of myself today because
_____

One thing I can improve upon tomorrow is
_____

What is my biggest struggle right now?
_____

Who can I ask to support me with this?
_____

What is my main goal this week?
_____

What does my idea of success look like next week?
_____
_____
_____

What three daily actions can I take to reach that goal?

1. _____
   _____
2. _____
   _____
3. _____
   _____

> **Quick Tip**
>
> Sometimes, it's tempting to focus on one thing as the root of our health issues. The human body is a complex system, with nothing working in isolation. By looking at all aspects of our lives, we can pinpoint areas contributing to illness. At this point, you do not need to jump in and change everything overnight. Just be aware of what aspects of your lifestyle could do with a little tweak. Write down which of the six lifestyle factors you want to improve. We'll get to them later.

The healthy lifestyle pillar I will improve first is

_____

CHAPTER 4: What Diseases Can This Program Help?

"If the truth be known, coronary artery disease is a toothless paper tiger that need never exist, and if it does exist, it need never ever progress."
Dr Caldwell Esselstyn.

What's In This Chapter?

In this chapter, I'll fill your brain with science. We'll discuss specific disease states and how they relate to lifestyle. I'll provide evidence that supports whole plant food nutrition to prevent, treat, and possibly reverse each disease. Get ready to have your mind blown!

It is essential to understand that all the science in the world cannot account for your personal situation. I said this at the start of the book, and I'll repeat myself now: I am not a doctor. Do not follow my advice without consulting your primary care physician or specialist. Use the following information as a knowledge base to discuss your treatment options with your medical team.

> **Note:** Meta-analyses and systematic reviews combine evidence from many individual studies. They are considered the highest-quality and most robust form of scientific evidence because they examine results from different scientists who study the same topic. I'll share some with you in this chapter.

Cancer

Cancer is the leading cause of death worldwide, accounting for ten million deaths annually as of 2020. According to the World Health Organization, a third of all cancer deaths are due to five risks: smoking, high body mass index (obesity), low fruit and vegetable intake, lack of exercise, and alcohol consumption [14].

The body is continuously recycling itself. Old cells die and are broken down into constituent parts to be remade into new ones. Every second, millions of DNA molecules in our bodies are being replicated, making new proteins. Sometimes, this replication process goes awry, and the systems that identify and fix errors fail to correct the problems. This is the beginning of cancer. Cancer occurs when malignant cells in the body don't die. Instead, they keep growing at the expense of the body's vital organs.

Why does this occur? Cancer does not have just one cause. Oxidative damage, chemical toxins, virus exposure, radiation and food can mutate cells. You may be surprised that only 5-10% of cancers are genetically based, leaving 90-95% largely within our control [15]. Even if only half of all cancers were caused by lifestyle factors, wouldn't you want to do everything you could to avoid them? Let's take a look at some research.

Meat

In the 1980s, nutritional biochemist Dr. T Collin Campbell travelled to China to compare the diets of plant-based eaters with meat eaters. He found that the more meat people consumed, the more cancer they developed [16]. He documented his findings in the book The China Study, which has since become one of the most important books about nutrition and chronic disease risk ever written and a mainstay for every plant-based enthusiast.

Common cancers associated with eating animal protein include cancer of the gastrointestinal tract, colon, mouth, breast, pancreas, prostate and bladder [15].

In 2018, the International Agency for Research on Cancer, part of the World Health Organization, released a report on red and processed meat. The report stated that red meat was probably carcinogenic to humans and classified it as a Group 2A carcinogen. Glyphosate, malathion, and lead are also in this group. It also classified processed meat, such as sliced deli meats, salami, bacon, sausage, and hot dogs, as a Group 1 carcinogen [17]. Group 1 carcinogens include formaldehyde, asbestos, aflatoxins, benzene, and tobacco.

> If you don't remember anything from this book, remember this. Meat is carcinogenic.

Dairy

Breast cancer is the most common cancer affecting women in the USA, and the incidence of the disease continues to grow globally. There is conflicting research about the benefits of dairy products to human health. Studies have shown that people who eat high-fat dairy products are at a greater risk of developing breast cancer [18] and that people who eat no dairy at all have the lowest risk [19]. Certainly, countries with high soy consumption have lower incidences of breast cancer. Is that because of soy's protective qualities or the lack of dairy consumption? It's most likely both.

It's not just women who are at risk of cancer from eating dairy products. A 2022 study looking at the diets of 28000 men found that those who eat 430 gm (about 1 ½ cups) of dairy daily were at a 60% increased risk of developing prostate cancer compared to men who ate no dairy foods [20].

A Quick Word About Soy

What about soy? Doesn't soy give you breast cancer? Don't men get man-boobs from soy? Nothing could be further from the truth. That myth was perpetuated by Men's Health magazine back in 2009 and retracted in 2019 [21]. It's just pure fiction. A 2021 review of 149 research studies concluded that there was little evidence that soy foods exert untoward effects on adults [22].

Soy contains phyto (plant) chemicals called phytoestrogens. Isoflavones, are a type of phytoestrogen. They are unlike human or animal estrogens and they don't have the same effect on the human body, even though they have similar chemical structures. Soy has antioxidant qualities; it can protect against both breast and prostate cancer, increase bone mineral density, and protect against cognitive decline [23].

So where do man boobs come from if not from soy? The medical term for man boobs is gynecomastia and relates to the enlarged breast gland tissue in men and boys. It's caused by a lack of testosterone and an excess of estrogen hormones. Animal estrogen hormones can be ingested by eating dairy and animal products. So, if man boobs are a concern, look first to the animal-based estrogens in the diet.

Ultra-processed Food

Up to 60% of all calories consumed in high and medium-income countries (i.e., the Western World) come from ultra-processed foods. Ultra-processed foods are convenient, ready-to-eat foods containing additives not typically found in the home kitchen.

The European Prospective Investigation into Cancer and Nutrition (EPIC) gathered nutrition data from over a quarter of a million people from seven European countries over eleven years. They found that people who regularly eat ultra-processed foods such as sugar-sweetened beverages and processed animal products are at increased risk of cancer and other lifestyle-based diseases, including cardiovascular disease and diabetes [24].

Preventing Cancer

In 2007, the World Cancer Research Fund and the American Institute of Cancer Research released eight lifestyle recommendations for cancer prevention. They are: maintain lean body weight, be physically active, limit energy-dense foods and sugary drinks, eat foods of plant origin, limit red and processed meat, limit alcohol, limit salt, avoid moldy grains and legumes, and meet nutritional needs through diet, not added supplements.

Researchers followed 30,000 post-menopausal women for 7 years. The women following just three of these recommendations, eating a plant-based diet, limiting alcohol, and maintaining a lean body weight, had 62% less incidence of developing breast cancer than the women who did not [25]. One mechanism that may be attributable to reduced breast cancer risk is fiber. A 2020 meta-analysis of twenty studies found that eating more fiber reduces the risk of developing breast cancer [26].

It's not just breast cancer that takes a hit with fiber consumption. Many cancers can be prevented by adding more fiber to your diet, including colorectal, pancreatic, gastrointestinal, ovarian, and renal cancers, to name a few [27].

What is it about plant-based foods that makes them so good at preventing cancer from forming? Phytonutrients (plant nutrients), including antioxidants, have powerful anti-cancer properties. They can reduce DNA damage and scavenge nasty molecules called reactive oxygen species (ROS). As far back as 1981, a study proposed that as many as 80% of all cancers could be prevented by increased fruit and vegetable intake [28]. This study focused on a class of phytonutrients called carotenoids found in carrots, sweet potatoes, pumpkin, grapefruit, bell peppers, leafy greens, tomatoes, and broccoli. Since then, we have learned that the whole food, not the isolated nutrients, has the cancer-fighting properties and that supplementing with carotenoids is ineffective. Here's a few examples:

Resveratrol, found in the skin of grapes and berries, exhibits anticancer properties against various tumors, including lymphoid and myeloid cancers, multiple myeloma, and cancers of the breast, prostate, stomach, colon, and pancreas [29].

Quercetin, found in green tea, berries and leafy greens, has been shown to inhibit inflammation and prevent colon and lung cancer [30].

Sulforaphane found in cruciferous vegetables such as broccoli acts via many cellular mechanisms to stop cancer in its tracks [31]. Head to Chapter 6 to find out more about the amazing benefits of phytonutrients.

Diabetes

Diabetes results from the hormone insulin's inability to allow glucose into a cell. The pancreas, the organ that produces insulin, either stops producing the hormone or does not produce enough insulin. Insulin resistance, whereby the insulin produced cannot be utilized by the cells, is a precursor to diabetes and is often called *pre-diabetes*.

There are many types of diabetes. The most common diabetes type is type 2 – it represents over 90% of all diabetes cases [32]. Diabetes killed 3.4 million people in 2024. That is one person every six seconds. By 2050 the International Diabetes Federation estimates 853 million people (13% of the population) will have diabetes. This has to stop. Let's find out why people are developing diabetes.

Type 2 Diabetes

Type 2 diabetes was once called *adult-onset diabetes* because it generally occurs in older adults. However, today, even children are developing type 2 diabetes. Why? Because they are carrying excess body fat.

Think of a muscle cell, for example, as an engine room. The engine's fuel is glucose, which needs to get into the engine room to run the engine (your body). The door to the engine room is locked, and insulin is the key that opens the door to let in the glucose. In the case of type 2 diabetes, the lock is clogged up with fat, so the insulin key will not work. The door won't open, so the glucose can't fuel the engine. The glucose floats around in the blood, causing havoc to the blood vessels. Meanwhile, the engine has no fuel, so it doesn't run properly. It's not the glucose's fault that it can't get into the cell. The reason it can't get into the cell is because the cell is full of FAT!

Some people think that diabetes is all about sugar. To an extent, sugar is involved, but the primary determinant of type 2 diabetes is fat. Excess fat creates inflammation that leads to insulin resistance and type 2 diabetes. It sounds overly simple, but losing fat is a great way to prevent and possibly reverse diabetes. Think about where the fat comes from in your diet. Animal products, pastries, snack foods, cheese, ice cream, fried foods, fast food, ready meals, restaurant meals, and snack foods.

Reducing body fat by just 7% can prevent type 2 diabetes [5]. Oh, and did I tell you that whenever insulin is released, fat burning stops, and fat storage activates?

A UK study enrolled 306 people from 49 different diabetes clinics. It separated half of them into a control group (where they received the usual diabetes care) and the other half into an intervention group. The intervention group was given a low-calorie diet to help them lose weight. After 12 months, 86%

of the people in the intervention group who had lost 15kg (33lb) reversed their diabetes altogether. Even the people who lost less weight had great results. Remission was achieved by 34% of people who lost between 5-10 kg (11-22 lb) and by 57% of those who lost between 10 – 15 kg (22 – 33 lb) [33]. This shows that you don't need to be a weight loss superstar to improve your diabetes. Every kilo lost counts.

Type 1 Diabetes

Type 1 diabetes is completely different. It's an autoimmune disease whereby the pancreatic cells that produce insulin, the beta cells, die. So, even though the lock to the metaphorical engine room may be clear and ready to let glucose inside, there is no insulin key. So, the glucose still can't get in to fuel the engine. You may say, "Well, just pump some insulin in," – and that is precisely what people with type 1 diabetes do. They inject themselves daily (and usually multiple times per day) with insulin. Type 1 diabetes requires constant monitoring of glucose which can be a tremendous burden. Sometimes, getting the exact amount of insulin is challenging, which can cause complications.

One of the ways to lessen the burden of type 1 diabetes is with nutrition. A whole plant foods diet can improve glycemic control, increase insulin sensitivity, and reduce medication needs in people with type 1 diabetes. In a 2024 study that assigned people with type 1 diabetes to a whole plant foods diet, in just 12 weeks, insulin requirements decreased by 24% [34]. As a bonus, participants lost 5.2 kg (11.5 lb), and their HbA1c (an indicator of diabetes status) decreased by 0.8%. This is fantastic news because, for a long time, people thought that diet had nothing to do with type 1 diabetes. I'm glad to report that it does.

Gestational Diabetes

Gestational diabetes can occur in some pregnant women. When pregnant, the body makes hormones at maximum capacity; sometimes, the pancreas can't keep up. Having gestational diabetes can be a risk factor for both the baby and mother to develop type 2 diabetes. Up to 50% of woman with gestational diabetes will go on to develop type 2 diabetes after giving birth [35]. Gestational diabetes can also make the fetus grow too big for a vaginal birth [36]. It often has no symptoms, so it is vital to maintain regular obstetric consultations during pregnancy to make sure all is well. If you do have gestational diabetes, it usually resolves itself after your baby is born. However, to ensure that diabetes does not rear its ugly head later on, it's best to reach a healthy body weight after delivery.

Alzheimer's disease

Alzheimer's disease is a type of cognitive decline that first affects memory and can progress to confusion, personality changes, mood swings, and loss of inhibition. In the end stages of the disease, people may not recognize their family members or their environment. Presently, there is no cure for Alzheimer's disease.

While writing this book, Dr. Dean Ornish, a renowned lifestyle physician, published the results of a lifestyle intervention for people diagnosed with mild Alzheimer's disease. The multidimensional program, featuring plant-based nutrition, showed marked improvement in cognition and brain function and slowed the progression of Alzheimer's disease. Participants in the control group who did not receive the intervention got worse [37]. While genetics can play a part in Alzheimer's disease [38], this trial shows that lifestyle can arrest its progression.

Alzheimer's disease is also closely linked to diabetes. It is often referred to as type 3 diabetes or diabetes of the brain. Up to 80% of people diagnosed with Alzheimer's disease also have diabetes [39]. The brain uses up a whole heap of glucose to function. Even though the brain only weighs 2% of your body weight, it uses up 25% of the glucose! So, when there is glucose dysfunction, it affects the brain.

High Cholesterol (Dyslipidemia)

Dyslipidemia is a sciencey way of saying too much blood cholesterol. Your body makes its own cholesterol. If you eat too much saturated fat from meat, dairy, palm and olive oils, this can raise your blood cholesterol. High cholesterol is a risk factor for heart disease, high blood pressure, and stroke. There are different measures of cholesterol that you can become familiar with.

Total Cholesterol

Total cholesterol is a measure of all the different cholesterols that circulate in your blood. Generally, doctors like to see total cholesterol below 200 mg/dL (5.18 mmol/L), however the latest guidelines from the Centers for Disease Control suggest keeping total cholesterol below 150 mg/dL (3.88 mmol/L) [40].

In Europe, there is not a one-size-fits-all approach. Depending upon other risk factors including age, gender, blood pressure, diabetes and smoking status, optimal total cholesterol targets vary [41].

Each cholesterol molecule measured in the blood attaches to a lipoprotein and is described based on its size and density. The different sized cholesterol molecules are described next.

HDL-Cholesterol

HDL-c is high-density lipoprotein cholesterol, which some call the 'good' cholesterol. Normal ranges are 35–65 mg/dL (0.9–1.7 mmol/L) for men and 35–80 mg/dL (0.9–2.1 mol/L) for women. HDL cholesterol helps remove other cholesterol from the blood and sends it back to the liver for recycling. HDL cholesterol levels within the normal range lessen your heart disease and stroke risk.

LDL-Cholesterol

LDL-c stands for low-density lipoprotein cholesterol. Some call this the 'bad' cholesterol. The normal range for LDL-c is under 100 mg/dL (2.59 mmol/L). Animal products contain cholesterol, but plants do not. So, switching from an animal-based diet to a whole plant foods diet is a great way to decrease both saturated fat and dietary cholesterol.

Important Cholesterol Numbers

Ideal Cholesterol Targets (CDC) [40]	
Total Cholesterol	< 150 mg/dL
LDL Cholesterol	< 100 mg/dL
HDL Cholesterol	> 40 mg/dL (Male) > 50 mg/dL (Female)
Triglycerides	<150 mg/dL

Atherosclerosis

Atherosclerosis is the process by which too much circulating LDL cholesterol gets stuck inside blood vessels, causing hardening, narrowing (stenosis), and blockages. It's a complex process that I will try to simplify.

Circulating LDL cholesterol molecules can irritate the insides of blood vessel walls, called the endothelium, and get stuck. The immune system sends in the cavalry (macrophages), which gobble up the LDL cholesterol and form a fatty streak. If you are still eating the same way that caused the assault, this fatty streak can form a fibrous plaque that can reduce the diameter of the blood vessel. Remember, blood is still pumping past this plaque every second. This friction can cause the plaque to rupture, forming a thrombus (blood clot) that can block the blood vessel. Blockages in blood vessels restrict blood flow, causing tissue damage and death (necrosis) downstream of the blockage.

Atherosclerosis is the cause of heart attacks, strokes, peripheral artery disease, and vascular dementia.

Atherosclerosis is entirely reversible—not through stents and bypass surgeries, but through diet. Consuming saturated fat creates an environment that promotes the formation of atherosclerosis, so removing saturated fat and switching to a whole plant foods diet can reverse the disease.

Lowering LDL cholesterol to 50−70 mg/dL (1.3−1.8 mmol/L) creates an environment in the arteries that cannot form atherosclerotic plaque [42].

Heart Disease

High cholesterol and heart disease are incredibly connected. The type of heart disease that kills one in five people is called coronary artery disease. It is the disease that gives people heart attacks, like the one that killed my dad. If there is one place you don't want to have atherosclerosis, it's in the arteries that feed the heart.

Way back in 1990, two years before my dad died, Dr. Dean Ornish sought to find out what would happen if he changed the diets of people with existing heart disease [43]. For one year, he asked 28 patients (the intervention group) to eat a low-fat plant-based diet and participate in stress management, exercise, and smoking cessation. He had another 20 patients (the control group) follow the usual care offered to heart disease patients at the time. After one year, the intervention group saw the following improvements:

- Total cholesterol dropped by 24.3%
- LDL cholesterol dropped by 37.4%
- Angina frequency dropped by 91%, duration by 42%, and severity by 28%. Angina is pain in the chest caused by decreased blood flow to the heart.
- Coronary artery stenosis (narrowing) dropped from 40%−37.8%. This may not seem like a lot, but blood vessels are cylinders, and increasing their diameter can exponentially increase blood flow.

A vital factor to remember is that the intervention followed what scientists call a 'dose-dependent' relationship. This means the more closely a person followed the diet, the more heart disease reversal they experienced.

You may wonder what happened to the 20 people who followed the usual medical care advice.

- Angina frequency increased by 165%, angina duration increased by 95%, and angina severity increased by 39%.
- Coronary artery stenosis increased from 42.7% to 46.1%. This means the arteries feeding the heart became even more blocked.

The control group ended up with worse heart disease a year later. I'm not sure about you, but I would expect my doctor to help me reduce my heart disease, not make it worse. This just shows how out-of-touch general medical advice for heart disease was in 1990. Following general medical guidelines is not a cure, but eating plants is.

Since then, Dr. Ornish has created the only lifestyle program in the USA covered by health insurance that can reverse heart disease without medications or surgery. For details on the Ornish program, see the resources section at the back of the book.

Dr. Caldwell Esselstyn is another US doctor who used a low-fat plant-based diet to treat his patients with heart disease [44]. He prescribed the diet to 198 consecutive patients with existing heart disease and other comorbidities, including high blood pressure, high cholesterol, and diabetes. He followed each of them for about four years. Of the 177 patients who followed the diet, thirty-nine experienced complete disease reversal. At the start of the study 112 people in the intervention group had angina symptoms. By the end of the study, 104 of them had reduced symptoms or had no angina at all. The average weight loss for those who followed the diet was 18.7lb (8.5kg).

What happened to the 21 people who did not follow Dr. Esselstyn's advice to eat a low-fat, plant-based diet? Two of them died of heart attacks. One had a heart transplant, two had strokes, four needed stents, three had bypass surgery, and one had the plaque sucked out of their arteries. You do not need to be a mathematician to see that the intervention was a resounding success.

High blood pressure (Hypertension)

High blood pressure (hypertension) is a warning sign of worse things to come. Hypertension can be a precursor to heart disease, stroke, dementia, vision loss, and atherosclerosis. Over 1.4 billion people are walking around with high blood pressure, and it kills 9 million people per year globally [45].

Half of the people with high blood pressure do not know it because it usually has no symptoms. To combat the naivety of high blood pressure, doctors recommend people buy a home blood pressure monitor and take regular readings. I take my blood pressure often to know where I'm at. I have a family history of high blood pressure, and knowing that I'm doing everything in my power to keep it within normal ranges gives me peace of mind.

Home blood pressure monitors are inexpensive, easy to use, and non-invasive. If you have ever had a high blood pressure reading at your doctor's office, I urge you to monitor your blood pressure at home regularly.

There are two readings for blood pressure:

- Systolic blood pressure is the pressure upon the artery walls when the heart pumps blood. Healthy systolic blood pressure is <120 mmHg (millimeters of mercury).

- Diastolic blood pressure is the pressure exerted upon the artery walls when the heart rests between beats and fills with blood. Healthy diastolic blood pressure is <80 mmHg (millimeters of mercury).

Different countries have different definitions of hypertension, but a consistent blood pressure of 120/80 mmHg can reduce the risk of cardiovascular events and death [46].

USA [47]			Europe [48]		
Risk	Systolic	Diastolic	Risk	Systolic	Diastolic
			Optimal	Below 120	Below 80
Normal	Below 120	Below 80	Normal	120-129	80-84
Elevated	120-129	Below 80	High Normal	130-139	85-89
Hypertension Stage 1	130-139	80-89	Grade1 Hypertension	140-159	90-99
Hypertension Stage 2	140 or more	90 or more	Grade 2 Hypertension	160-179	100-109
Crisis Hypertension	180 or more	120 or more	Grade 3 Hypertension	180 or more	110 or more

All numbers above represent millimeters of mercury.

How can you keep your blood pressure within normal ranges? Let's take a look.

Exercise

Chapter 3 discussed the effect of exercise on blood pressure. If you haven't read it yet, please do so now. I want to stress the importance of exercise to health again. As we continue this journey together, I will also emphasize the importance of physical activity in combating other conditions.

A meta-analysis from 2022 analyzed twenty-four studies that examined the effect of exercise on hypertension. It found that 20—60 minutes of vigorous aerobic exercise done 3—4 times per week can reduce systolic blood pressure by 10 mmHg and diastolic blood pressure by 6 mmHg [49]. This is as good a result as you could expect from some medications.

The important thing to stress is that exercise needs to be a lifelong pursuit. Anyone can exercise for a month or two, but exercise needs to be part of your weekly routine for lasting health and lower blood pressure. Additionally, when exercise is accompanied by weight loss, the benefits to blood pressure are even better.

Salt

Have you heard of the DASH diet? It's widely studied and stands for Dietary Approach to Stop Hypertension. It works. Following the DASH principles of eating more plant foods, fewer animal products and fewer ultra-processed foods can lower blood pressure. One reason the DASH diet works is that it limits sodium, which is found in table salt, restaurant food, ready meals, and ultra-processed foods.

Sodium raises blood pressure because it is best friends with water. It makes the body hold onto water, creating a greater blood volume that exerts more pressure on the arterial walls. This extra fluid also stresses the kidneys, which must filter it. Not surprisingly, eating less sodium has the opposite effect. It lowers blood pressure, reduces edema (water retention), and keeps the kidneys happy.

A meta-analysis with a combined population of over 1.3 million people found that the more DASH-like their diet, the less risk of death [50]. Awesome!

If you are unsure about the optimal amount of sodium for a healthy diet, look at the labels on packaged foods. If the amount of sodium (in mg) is more than the number of calories per serve, the food has too much sodium.

Food and Blood Pressure

Losing weight can lower blood pressure considerably. A meta-analysis of twenty-five studies found that every kilogram of weight loss lowers systolic blood pressure by 1mmHg [51]. I'll discuss weight loss in the next section.

Certain foods can lower blood pressure. These include beets and leafy green vegetables. What is in these foods that help lower blood pressure? Nitrates.

Nitrates are vasodilators. That means they help relax blood vessels so they widen and allow blood to flow easily. To lower systolic blood pressure by about 5mmHg, the optimum dose of beet juice is 70-250 ml daily [52]. This is 100% beet juice made at home, not beet-flavored sugar drinks.

Leafy greens are power packed with nitrates. Try them all: kale, collards, spinach, rocket (arugula), Swiss chard (silverbeet). Find the ones you like the best. My husband dislikes kale. He must be an alien! I don't try to sneak kale into his food – that would be mean. Instead, I find greens he likes, such as spinach and arugula, and we eat them instead. I eat kale when I'm making food just for myself.

The effect of greens on blood pressure follows a dose-response. Do you remember what that means? It means the more greens you eat, the lower your blood pressure. Score!

Garlic lowers blood pressure, too, so does taking garlic supplements, as long as the only ingredient in the supplement is powdered garlic. Eating or taking the equivalent of two cloves of garlic per day for at least 12 weeks can lower systolic blood pressure by over 8 mmHg and diastolic blood pressure by 6 mmHg [53]. These results are for people with already high blood pressure. People with normal blood pressure won't see such impressive results. Hey – if you have normal blood pressure, you don't need to lower it; just keep it healthy. Even if you don't like the taste of garlic in your food, taking a supplement might be an alternative.

Hibiscus tea also gets an A+ in the blood pressure-lowering class. But it needs to be strong, and you must drink it daily. Two cups of strong hibiscus tea made with water (no sweetener) daily can have the same blood pressure-lowering effect as low-dose medication [54].

I promote a whole plant foods diet for optimal health in this book. Let's examine the science behind this diet and its effect on blood pressure.

A study using the data of 11,000 people from the Oxford University European Prospective Investigation into Cancer and Nutrition (EPIC-Oxford) found that plant-based eaters are less likely to have high blood pressure than meat eaters [55]. Even if they don't have diagnosed hypertension, vegans across the board have lower blood pressure than meat eaters.

Are you wondering why you should care about your blood pressure? High blood pressure is a risk factor for other diseases. And Death. Yes, Death with a capital D. Lowering your systolic blood pressure by just 5 mmHg can reduce your risk of stroke by 14%, your risk of heart attack by 9%, and your overall risk of untimely death by 7% [56]. Those are pretty good reasons to keep your blood pressure in the normal range.

Make a quick note of all the blood pressure-lowering foods you want to add to your diet.

_____

_____

_____

_____

_____

Stress

Some stress is good stress. For example, when you are running to catch the bus, your heart is pumping to get all that oxygenated blood to your muscles, and once you are on the bus, you calm down. Your heart rate returns to normal, and the stress subsides.

But what if it doesn't? What if you are on the bus but worried about the meeting with your boss? Or you fought with your partner and can't get it out of your mind? This is chronic stress. It can be caused by, well, life. Chronic stress keeps your heart rate high, your blood pressure high, and your anxiety levels high. It is not good for you at all.

Removing chronic stress from your life is imperative for your health. I could write another book on ways to alleviate stress. If you think you are under stress, take it seriously. Don't sweep it under the rug. Don't ignore it and hope the stress will go away. Deal with it, however that might look for you.

If you need to have serious conversations with people in your life about how their actions affect you, then have those conversations. If you need to remove yourself from an escalating situation, do so. If you need to walk out of a room and take five deep breaths, then do that. Short-term solutions such as deep breathing work in the moment, but chronic stress affects all parts of your life and must be addressed seriously.

Here are some ideas to help you reduce your stress:

- Talk to someone. A therapist, a counselor, a friend or relative. A burden shared is a burden halved.

- Exercise – get your frustrations out with sweat.
- Try relaxation exercises such as deep breathing, meditation, tai-chi, or yoga.
- Download and use an app such as Calm® or Headspace®.
- Garden, knit, walk the dog – do whatever makes you happy and helps clear your head.
- Get out in nature. Leave the world behind and head to the forest or the ocean. Feel the wind in your hair and the sun on your skin. Breathe the fresh air.

Many people turn to sweet, salty, or oily foods to cope with stress. Before you put your hand in the cookie jar or order a double fudge sundae, try one of the suggestions above. Your body will thank you.

These are suggestions that you can try for yourself. If you find that your emotions are out of control or you can't manage your stress, please seek professional help.

Obesity

Obesity is defined as having a body mass index (BMI) greater than 30. This number is determined by dividing your weight in kilograms by your height in meters squared. For example, I'm 1.73m tall and I weigh 70kg. So, my BMI is $70/(1.73)^2 = 23.4$. The normal BMI range is 19-25. Overweight BMI is 26-29.

Obesity is the epidemic of the 21st century. In the USA, at the time of writing this book, 74% of Americans are overweight and 42% are obese [57]. It's a similar story in the UK, where 64% of adults are overweight and 26% are obese [58], and Australia with 66% overweight and 32% obese [59]. When you read this book, I doubt those numbers will be lower.

Almost all my clients want to lose weight. The modern food system has made it very easy for people to become obese. High-fat, high-sugar, and high-calorie foods are all around us. There are no warning labels to tell us the products are unhealthy. Even when they think they are eating healthily, it's hard to stay at a healthy weight when the environment is working against them. Just walk into any food court in any mall in the world. If you are lucky, there may be one healthy option. The rest is junk!

Obesity is a disease unto itself and is also a risk factor for many other diseases. Obesity increases the risk of heart disease, diabetes, rheumatoid arthritis, dementia, and cancer, to name a few.

In addition, obesity accelerates aging at the level of our DNA. Telomeres are the end strands of DNA. Researchers describe them as being like the ends of a shoelace. They help keep the DNA together. Over time, they shorten, causing cell death and aging. For every BMI point (kg/m^2) over 25, telomere shortening is equivalent to aging one year [60]. For example, if you are 45 and have a BMI of 35, your biological age is 55. In case you didn't understand the math: 35 (your BMI) minus 25 (normal BMI) = 10. Add the 10 to your age, and you get 55. This is another reason to maintain your weight in the normal BMI range.

Switching to a whole plant foods diet from a standard Western eating pattern is the best way to resolve obesity and, in turn, resolve other health complications related to it.

The BROAD study was a trial conducted in New Zealand whereby people with obesity and one other metabolic complication were placed on a whole food plant-based diet for 12 weeks. Researchers then followed up after six and 12 months. During the trial, people lost an average of 12 kg (26 lb), reducing their BMI by 4 points [61]. Let's put that into perspective. Obesity is defined as a BMI >30, whilst a healthy BMI is 19-25. This study shows that in just a few months, obesity can almost be reversed. If the subjects of this intervention continued to eat a whole plant foods diet, they would likely lose the remaining weight to put them in a healthy BMI range.

Researchers tested other parameters, too, and reductions in cholesterol, medications, and diabetes accompanied the weight loss. They also asked people about how they felt. At six months, people eating the whole food plant-based diet reported: "an increased quality of life, general and nutritional self-efficacy, and self-esteem, without significant changes in food enjoyment, cost or exercise." How good is that! People felt better, had more confidence, and didn't feel like they were missing out or made to do extra exercise. That's a win-win. Oh—and it wasn't more expensive to eat this way. I'll talk about the cost of eating whole plant foods in Chapter 16.

Being overweight or obese affects people in so many ways. It is much more than not being able to fit into favorite clothes or liking what they see in the mirror. Obesity stops people from living their lives to the fullest.

I love downhill skiing. Whilst it is entirely possible to ski when obese, I rarely see obese people on the mountain. Is that because obese people like doing other things? Maybe. Or is that because their obesity is holding them back from trying new things? Granted, even normal-weight people should not just go downhill skiing without proper training and a base fitness level, but I hope you get my point. Does obesity stop people from getting fit, or do people become obese because they don't exercise?

What I'm trying to say here is that obesity is multifaceted. If you suffer from this disease state (yes, it's a disease), you may be fixated on the scale, determined to lose pounds. Whilst losing weight can lower your risk of other diseases [62], including cardiovascular disease and diabetes, focusing solely on weight loss can be a rollercoaster of emotions and detrimental to long-term mental health. Instead of targeting weight loss as an ultimate goal, focus on the daily habits that help you reach your optimal weight. How can you make your next meal as healthy as possible? How can you incorporate more movement into your day? How can you get more restorative sleep? Focus on habit building, which results in weight loss—if that is what your body needs. Chapter 20 is all about creating healthy habits. Don't go there yet, there's lots to learn first.

Metabolic Syndrome

The metabolic syndrome is a group of symptoms that alerts doctors and patients that work needs to be done to improve health. If you have higher than normal cholesterol, blood pressure, HbA1c, or any of your blood chemistry numbers are out of normal range, it's time to take lifestyle change seriously. To be considered as having metabolic syndrome, you need to have three of the following five symptoms [63].

1. **Visceral adiposity** (central fatness)—waist circumference greater than 40 inches (101cm) for men and 35 inches (89cm) for women. This is an indication of excess fat in and around vital organs.
2. **Insulin resistance**—fasting blood glucose ≥100 mg/dL (5.5 mmol/L) or on medication to lower glucose. This is considered pre-diabetes.
3. **Dyslipidemia (low HDL cholesterol)** <40 mg/dL (1.0 mmol/L) for men and <50 mg/dL (1.3 mmol/L) for women, or on cholesterol medications.
4. **High triglycerides** ≥150 mg/dL (1.7 mmol/L).
5. **Hypertension (high blood pressure)** >130mmHg (systolic) or >85mmHg (diastolic), or on blood pressure lowering medication.

It is essential to see your primary care physician at least once per year to have a complete check-up, including blood work, so that you know your numbers. Knowing where you stand can save your life. If you have not been to the doctor to find out this information in more than twelve months, even if you feel fine, drop this book right now and make an appointment. Knowledge is power. If you know, then you can take action.

These are your starting numbers. If any of your numbers are not what you had hoped for, you can start implementing healthy lifestyle habits immediately and check them again in a few months.

Inflammation

If you have ever been on WebMD® or other internet medical websites, you would have read about inflammation being the root cause of many lifestyle diseases. But what is it?

Acute inflammation occurs when you are injured. If you fall over and bang your knee, it might swell and be tender to the touch. The body senses the injury and immediately dilates the blood vessels around the injury, sending more blood and heat to the injury site. Then, leukocytes (white blood cells) are dispatched to clean up microorganisms, damaged tissues, and other debris. Macrophages (big eaters) are then employed to eat up the damaged tissue and recycle it into the bloodstream by a process called phagocytosis. This is healing. After a time, the body returns to a pre-injured state.

Chronic inflammation, however, is an ongoing inflammatory response without acute injury. In essence, the body is constantly attacking itself. It can occur from long-term exposure to chemicals, an autoimmune disorder, oxidative stress, mitochondrial dysfunction, or obesity. It can result in diabetes, arthritis, allergies, cardiovascular disease, hypertension, inflammatory bowel syndrome (IBS), Crohn's disease, fibromyalgia, liver disease, multiple sclerosis, and chronic obstructive pulmonary disease (COPD) [64].

Chronic inflammation is at the root of more deaths worldwide than any other cause. The World Health Organization ranks chronic inflammation as the greatest threat to world health. To avoid nasty chronic diseases, you should first lower your body's inflammatory response. But how do you do that? First, remove the cause of the inflammation.

One of the most significant effects (not the only effect) of inflammation comes from the gut. Heal your gut, and you will have less systemic inflammation. A starting point is to eat more fiber-rich fruit and vegetables while avoiding inflammatory foods.

Avoid foods that promote inflammation:

- Animal products, including processed and deli meats
- Dairy products – especially cheese
- Fats, oils, and fried foods
- Processed junk foods
- Chemical food additives, colors, and preservatives

What else promotes inflammation? Oxidative stress. This is when chemical toxins in our environment (either ingested, breathed in, or applied topically) cause damage to our cells, resulting in premature aging and cell damage, a precursor to cancer. To combat oxidative stress, one must first eliminate the toxins and introduce more antioxidants. Antioxidants stop oxidative stress in its tracks. Fresh fruit and vegetables have varying amounts of antioxidants, and eating them daily can have beneficial anti-inflammatory effects. The brighter and darker the veggies, the more antioxidants they have. Berries and darker fruits have increased antioxidant capacity, with higher concentrations in blueberries and wolfberries (goji berries).

Hormone Imbalances

To many, hormones and their effect on our bodies are a mystery. They go about their important jobs without us giving them a second thought. Insulin is a hormone that regulates blood glucose uptake into our cells. Thyroid hormones regulate metabolism. Growth hormones promote protein synthesis. Hormones are messenger molecules. They move through the bloodstream to their target tissue and get things done. But sometimes things can go awry.

Autoimmune Diseases

Hashimoto's

Hashimoto thyroiditis is a type of hypothyroidism, an autoimmune disorder whereby the thyroid gland is destroyed by the body's own immune cells. Five times as many women develop Hashimoto's than men. People with Hashimoto's are generally fatigued, have low blood pressure and a slow heart rate, can gain weight even in the absence of appetite, and can be intolerant to cold.

As an autoimmune condition, inflammation is at the root of Hashimoto's. A whole plant foods diet has the benefit of being anti-inflammatory by design. It's essential to have adequate intakes of iodine (seaweed is a good source—but not too much!), iron (green leafy vegetables, legumes, nuts, and seeds), selenium (Brazil nuts), protein (legumes, whole grains, vegetables, nuts, and seeds), unsaturated fatty acids (nuts and seeds) and fiber (vegetables, whole grains, legumes, fruit). As you can see, all the nutrients you need for a healthy thyroid gland can be found in wholesome plant foods.

Rheumatoid Arthritis

Rheumatoid arthritis is an autoimmune condition that affects the joints—usually of the hands and feet. Inflammation with the joint cavity damages the cartilage and the bone, making normal movement painful. Eventually, the joints can become deformed, making moving and using the hands difficult.

People with rheumatoid arthritis tend to have high cholesterol and are at greater risk of cardiovascular disease. Even though there is a strong genetic component to rheumatoid arthritis, this can be minimized or exacerbated by lifestyle factors. This means that even if you are genetically susceptible to developing rheumatoid arthritis, you can lessen your risk with a healthy lifestyle. Of course, the opposite is also true.

Losing weight is a great start. People who are overweight are three times more likely to develop rheumatoid arthritis than normal-weight individuals [65]. This is because fat cells produce inflammatory compounds called cytokines. The cytokine TNF-α (tumor necrosis factor-alpha) is a major player in the progression of rheumatoid arthritis. Being obese can reduce the effectiveness of anti-TNF-α drugs or other medications used to treat rheumatoid arthritis.

We already discussed how meat and fried foods increase inflammation, but a recent study has tested this with rheumatoid arthritis patients. A team in the Netherlands had arthritis patients try a plant-based diet for 16 weeks with fantastic results. Not only did the people see improvement in their arthritis symptoms, but they also lost weight, lowered their markers of inflammation, lowered their cholesterol, lowered their HbA1c (a marker of glucose control), and lowered their blood pressure [66]. When the researchers checked in on their patients a year later, they found that those on the plant-based diet continued to see improvements in their health. This shows how important it is to make lifestyle changes, not just short-term quick fixes.

Reproduction Problems

PCOS

Polycystic ovary syndrome (PCOS) is a hormone disorder affecting around 10% of women of childbearing age that can disrupt ovulation and fertility. PCOS can be very painful and debilitating. It is strongly connected to insulin resistance, and women with PCOS are at greater risk of developing type 2 diabetes. Symptoms include irregular periods, acne, hair loss or unusual hair growth, weight gain, and infertility—just to name a few. Diagnosis of PCOS requires the presence of at least two of the following: irregular periods, high androgen (male hormone) levels, or cystic ovaries.

As PCOS is related to insulin resistance, adopting an anti-inflammatory whole plant foods diet can be crucial in maintaining glucose control. The dark blue pigment in blueberries and pomegranates comes from a group of phytonutrients called anthocyanins, which have potent antioxidant and anti-inflammatory properties [67]. Soy foods (soy milk, edamame, tempeh, tofu, natto) contain isoflavone compounds called phytoestrogens.

These plant estrogens work with the body to lower the risk of cardiovascular disease, improve menopause symptoms, and decrease excess androgen hormones in women with PCOS [68].

> Dr. Nitu Bajekal has a fantastic book *Living PCOS Free*. I urge you to read it if you are suffering from PCOS or other female reproductive conditions.

Gut Issues

The human body contains ten times more microorganisms than human cells [69]. Think about that. People are more bacteria than humans. The gut is so crucial to overall health. When the gut microbiome (bacteria and other metabolites) is unhappy, your whole body is unhappy. The gut is integral to the immune system; it produces neurotransmitters such as serotonin, and there is direct communication between the microbiome and the brain. Having a healthy gut lowers inflammation and the risk of disease. Let's take a look at what happens when the gut is unhappy.

Ulcerative Colitis (UC) and Crohn's Disease

Ulcerative Colitis and Crohn's disease are different sides of the same coin. They are both characterized by inflammation and disruption of the gastrointestinal tract, causing pain, gas, difficulty with elimination, and diarrhea. If left unchecked, both ulcerative colitis and Crohn's disease may lead to colon cancer.

Ulcerative Colitis occurs usually only in the colon, whilst Crohn's disease can strike anywhere in the gastrointestinal tract from the mouth to the anus. In Crohn's disease, there may be healthy parts of the GI tract interspersed with areas of inflammation.

A Western diet high in saturated fat, animal products, and ultra-processed food is a breeding ground for inflammation and gut dysbiosis. Dysbiosis is a fancy way of saying there are too many 'bad' bacteria, not enough 'good' bacteria, and not enough variety of good bacteria for a healthy gut.

This diet pattern promotes the proliferation of harmful bacteria at the expense of good bacteria. In contrast, a plant-based diet high in vegetables, whole grains, legumes, and fruit is abundant in fiber. Fiber is the food that your good gut bacteria love. The more, the better. And the greater the variety, the better. Dr Will Bulsiewicz, in his book *Fiber Fueled*, says that the variety of plants eaten is the single most significant determinant of health.

You may have one of these conditions and be thinking, "There is no way I can eat all that fiber. It will worsen my symptoms!" You may be correct, in the short term at least. If your gastroenterologist has diagnosed you with either UC or Crohn's, speak to them about including more fiber-rich plant foods into your diet. There may be a period of adjustment. Some foods may not agree with you, but keep trying. Eventually, your gut will start to heal.

Irritable Bowel Syndrome

Irritable bowel syndrome is the general term for an upset gut. It may be the beginnings of UC or Crohn's disease, or you may have sensitivities to certain foods. For me, I know I cannot eat barley. It gives me a stomach ache and gas, and it is really uncomfortable. So I just don't eat it. I'm not worried that I can't eat barley because I can eat other whole grains like farro, wheat, oats, quinoa, and millet—so I know I'm not missing out on any nutrition.

If you can't eat any whole grains without discomfort or brassicas (broccoli, cabbage, cauliflower, kale) without bloating and gas, your gut may cry out for help. I urge you not to avoid all grains or greens in the quest for a pain-free existence. Instead, I encourage you to talk to your gastroenterologist to work out ways to increase the variety of plants you can tolerate.

You may have heard of the Low FODMAP diet researchers at Monash University in Australia created. FODMAP stands for Fermentable Oligosaccharides, Disaccharides, Monosaccharides And Polyols. These are all different types of carbohydrates. Foods including onions, eggplant, stone fruit, dairy products, high fructose corn syrup, and some beans and grains contain FODMAPs. Working with a registered dietician or nutritionist familiar with FODMAP elimination may be a way to alleviate gut distress.

It is important to note that the low-FODMAP diet was never intended to be a permanent lifestyle change. It was designed purely as a short-term intervention to identify specific foods that may be causing intestinal distress. Once those foods have been identified, under professional guidance, they may be reintroduced to the diet gradually. Eliminating whole food families (such as all grains or all stone fruit) is not gut-healthy.

For all gut-related issues, I recommend Dr Will Bulsiewicz's book, *Fiber Fueled*.

Workbook

Quiz

Answer True or False.

1. It doesn't matter what you eat; diabetes and heart disease are an inevitable part of aging.
2. The diet that can help prevent obesity is also the diet that can help prevent rheumatoid arthritis.
3. Blood pressure will lower by 1mmHg with every kilogram of weight loss.

ANSWERS in Appendix

Journal

Today I learned
___

Today I feel
___

I am proud of myself today because
___

One thing I can improve upon tomorrow is
___

What is my biggest struggle right now?
___

Who can I ask to support me with this?
___

What is my main goal this week?
___

What does my idea of success look like next week?
___
___
___
___

What three daily actions can I take to reach that goal?

1. _____
   _____

2. _____
   _____

3. _____
   _____

> **Quick Tip**
>
> You may have already ascertained that switching from a highly processed, animal-rich diet towards a whole plant foods diet can help with many metabolic complications and diseases. A whole plant foods diet may not be the magic cure for all ailments, but it is the best starting point. Once your diet is dialed in, you will have a clearer picture of your health and what you can do to help heal. For some people, change is immediate; for others, it takes time. Lean into it. Every step you take towards a more plant-centered existence is a step in the right direction.

CHAPTER 5: The Broken System

"When diet is wrong, medicine is of no use. When diet is correct, medicine is of no need." — Ayurvedic Proverb

What's In This Chapter?

In this chapter, you will learn why there are more people overweight or obese than normal weight in Western societies like the USA, the UK, and Australia. You will find out how the food industry manipulates you to buy their unhealthy products that make you sick.

Why Are We Fat?

Why are people fat? Why are people getting fatter? My grandparents and their friends weren't fat. If you look at pictures from the 1970s of people on the beach, why are there no fat people? Did they all stay at home? Or was the population thinner?

It turns out that the population was thinner. The US Centers for Disease Control and Prevention (CDC) only lets you see data from the past twenty years, but it is apparent that the population is getting fatter every year. The same applies to Australia, the UK, China, and Canada.

Hear me now. It's not your fault. I'll say it again.

IT'S NOT YOUR FAULT. (Sorry for shouting).

But why are people getting fat? Because the food system is broken. How many of us grow our own vegetables? How many of us mill our own flour? Or even walk to the store to buy it?

The supermarket is chock full of things in shiny packages and pretty boxes with unpronounceable ingredients. Foods with additives that are so addictive, they keep you coming back to buy more because they taste so good!

Additionally, industrialized farming means that store-bought veggies are missing some essential nutrients. The soil they are grown in is nutrient deficient, and the crops are sprayed with pesticides and herbicides. Phew! It's a sad state of affairs.

The Bliss Point

The food system is structured to make money for big corporations. The food companies don't care about your health; they care about money. Did you know you can go to university and get a degree in food science so you can devise ways to make food taste so good that people will keep buying it? There is a thing called the 'bliss point' that scientists have formulated to make you buy more of their products. The bliss point isn't just a happy accident— it's a carefully calculated formula designed to make food addictive. It is a perfect combination of sweet, salty, and fatty that is so delectable that the brain releases endorphins when the food is eaten.

Cue dopamine—the feel-good neurotransmitter that makes you want to return for seconds (and thirds). It's the same neural pathway that fuels drug addiction – except this time, it's not cocaine; it's chips or ice cream! Here's the kicker: Fat, sugar, and salt don't just taste good on their own. The combinations of all three together work synergistically to give your brain an even bigger hit, resulting in a bigger demand. The more you eat, the more you want. Food companies know this. Their goal is to obtain the bliss point for each food they produce, making stopping at just one bite nearly impossible. That feeling of "I just can't put this down". It's not a lack of self-control—it's by design.

These bliss point foods can trick your brain into ignoring your natural signals to stop eating. When you're stressed, upset, or bored, your brain goes straight for the chocolate or that extra-large bag of chips.

I believe this manipulation is borderline criminal. Innocent people like you are buying these foods, not knowing they could be contributing to serious illness. This is a system designed to undermine your health for profit.

You, however, will not be part of their evil plan. You will be healthy, handsome and gorgeous despite their fancy scientists, delicious bliss points, and shiny packaging. I challenge you to leave this corporate greed and move toward more whole, plant foods. Instead, support local organic farmers who give back to the earth and produce food of high nutrient density to fuel our bodies.

I urge you to omit all animal products. Scientific research has blamed ultra-processed foods and animal products for obesity and chronic disease. Here are just a few facts about meat and dairy.

1. Animal products contain saturated fat. Most plant foods (except palm oil and coconut) do not. Saturated fat sticks to the insides of your blood vessels and can cause atherosclerosis, heart disease [44], stroke, dementia [70, 71] and diabetes [72].

2. Animal products contain hormones that can harm our hormones, including promoting cancer [73].

3. Animal agriculture is not the same as it was fifty years ago. Animals eat genetically modified feed sprayed with pesticides, which get into their milk and muscles (meat). Animals are routinely fed antibiotics and other medications to make them grow faster. These synthetic chemicals, when ingested by the human body, can cause untold damage, including cancer [74].

4. Eggs and dairy foods contain cholesterol. Plant foods contain no cholesterol. Your body makes its own cholesterol. Extra cholesterol from animal products can lead to chronic diseases, including atherosclerosis and heart disease [75].

The Obesogenic Environment

Food Deserts

You might think you have complete control over what you eat unless you live in a food desert. A food desert is a geographical area with a distinct lack of healthy, affordable food. These areas don't lack food entirely (we're not talking about the barren Sahara here). There may be an abundance of food, but none is nutritionally sound. Some towns have multiple fast food outlets but nowhere to buy fresh fruit or vegetables. This is called a *food swamp*.

Think about the last time you drove from one city to another. Look out the window—what did you see? Every exit is a lineup of the usual suspects: a burger joint, a pizza place, a donut shop, and maybe a gas station stocked with sugary snacks. You can almost feel your arteries clogging as you pass.

Now, imagine living in a town where those outlets are your only option. Dollar stores and fast-food chains have conquered rural America, crowding the shelves with processed, chemical-laden food products. Where are the fresh fruit and vegetables? Some towns have two or three fast food options but not a single grocery store offering fresh, healthy food.

Food deserts and food swamps are often located in underserved minority communities with limited access to transportation [76]. It's not just a lack of options; it's a lack of access. When unhealthy food is all that is available and affordable, it's no surprise that people eat it. Willpower or personal choice have nothing to do with it—it's about survival.

In these areas, people are more likely to suffer from metabolic diseases, including obesity and cancer. A recent study found that American residents of food deserts and swamps were 77% more likely to die of obesity-related cancer than people with access to healthy food [77].

Marketing

The next time you step into your local supermarket, take a moment to really pay attention to how everything is carefully crafted to get you to spend more money. What sits right by the door? If it's around Easter, there's no escaping the mountains of chocolate. Swing by in June, and you're greeted with rows of hot dog buns and patriotic red, white, and blue sugar cookies. Come October, you can barely make it through the entrance without dodging stacks of Halloween candy. Temptation is everywhere, and let's face it—those cookies look delicious, don't they?

How can you resist tossing a pack (or two) into your cart before you've even made it to your grocery list? It does not stop there. Head down the aisles, and the deals hit you hard. Corn chips? Buy one, get one free. Soda? The two-liter bottle is cheaper than the smaller bottle. Have you noticed some cookie brands lately? They've exploded into seventeen different flavors, but you can't buy a small pack anymore. It's only family size. Why settle for a few when you can be nudged into buying a lot more?

The cold, hard truth is this: the food industry isn't looking out for your health. They're looking out for their bottom line.

USDA Guidelines

The USDA dietary guidelines are updated every five years. They tell Americans how to eat to maintain their health. They are also used to inform school nutrition and federal government nutrition programs. Most countries have their own set of dietary guidelines.

Hands up if you believe the dietary guidelines are based on the latest nutrition research? Yes, that's what I thought, too. Unfortunately, we are both wrong. A federal advisory committee looks at three pillars: scientific evidence, testimony from industry, and the public. This is where it gets murky. The food industry, particularly the livestock, egg, and dairy industries, has a lot of money and power. They make a lot of noise, which often drowns out science. Even when scientific evidence points to a whole plant foods diet as the healthiest, the guidelines will not reflect this because of industry influence. The meat, dairy, and egg industries will do whatever it takes to keep their products in the guidelines. There is not such a hullabaloo from the broccoli producers.

At the time of writing this book, the 2025 dietary guidelines are in the process of being updated. There are whispers that meat and dairy may start to take a back seat to plant foods. Only time will tell.

Government Subsidies

Why are eggs, dairy, and meat cheap, whilst fresh fruit and veggies are expensive? Many Western governments subsidize meat, egg, and dairy farmers to keep the prices of these commodities down. According to a 2023 report by the Environmental Working Group, a consumer watch organization, the USDA has handed out over $59 billion since 1995 to livestock producers. In contrast, the plant-based sector has received only $124 million since 2001 [78]. There is a lot of chatter on the internet about how expensive meat would be to the consumer if these subsidies were removed. Imagine how inexpensive fresh fruit and vegetables would be if the subsidies were given to crop farmers instead.

Workbook

Quiz

Answer True or False.

1. The main aim of food companies is to provide optimum nutrition to people.
2. The bliss point is a precise measure of sugar, fat, and salt that affects the brain to make food addictive.
3. If it weren't for government subsidies, buying meat would be a lot more expensive.
4. The USDA dietary guidelines are entirely based on scientific evidence to ensure the health of the nation.

ANSWERS in Appendix

Journal

Today I learned

Today I feel

I am proud of myself today because

One thing I can improve upon tomorrow is

What is my biggest struggle right now?

Who can I ask to support me with this?

What is my main goal this week?

What does my idea of success look like next week?

What three daily actions can I take to reach that goal?

1. _____
   _____

2. _____
   _____

3. _____
   _____

> **Quick Tip**
>
> I trust this chapter has made you more aware of all the forces working against you to improve your health. Once you know how the system works, you can be better informed to make the best decisions for you and your family. Open your eyes to the deception.

CHAPTER 6: Nutrition 101

"There are two types of cardiologists: those who are vegan and those who have not read the data." Dr Kim A Williams Sr., former American College of Cardiology president.

What's In This Chapter?

This chapter will give you a basic overview of nutrition science. It will cover macronutrients, micronutrients, and other important nutritional parts of whole foods. I will make this as easy to understand as possible. Don't worry if you don't understand everything in this chapter. You can use this chapter as a reference and refer back to it whenever you need.

Macronutrients

Macronutrients are literally BIG nutrients (as the word macro suggests). There are four macronutrients: carbohydrates, fat, protein, and alcohol. I'd like you to eliminate one of them from your diet.

Alcohol

Yes, I said it. If you want to be effortlessly slim and healthy for your entire life, there is no room for regular alcohol consumption. However, if you so desire to toast at a family wedding with a glass of bubbly once per year, I won't say anything. But, it is best for your health if you avoid regular alcohol consumption. A weekly drink is off limits, as is wine with dinner. Alcohol is a toxic drug, and it has no place in a healthy lifestyle.

Carbohydrates

NEWSFLASH!! CARBS ARE NOT YOUR ENEMY!!

Carbohydrates are not evil. Our bodies love them, and they are our preferred energy source. Carbohydrates are simply long chains of carbon and water molecules. They can be classified as simple carbohydrates (sugars) or complex carbohydrates (chains of sugars). Complex carbohydrates can be divided into two categories: starchy carbohydrates (like potatoes, rice, beans, and oatmeal) and non-starchy carbohydrates (like fruit, vegetables, and greens). This book encourages eating a lot of complex carbohydrates of both types.

What Is The Difference Between Simple And Complex Carbohydrates?

The human body loves sugar. The digestive system breaks down carbohydrate-based food into the simplest sugar, glucose, and uses that glucose to make energy for our bodies. Because complex carbohydrates are long chains of sugars, they take time to digest, so they are better for lasting energy and keeping you satisfied for longer. Complex carbohydrates from natural sources, including fresh fruit and vegetables, grains, and legumes, should make up the bulk of your diet.

When carbohydrates are processed into simple sugars, such as table sugar, corn syrup, processed sweets, or fizzy drinks (soda), they overload our system, giving us lots of energy but little nutrition. Simple sugars from bakery goods, candy, or sugary drinks get absorbed into the bloodstream quickly. They can give you a quick 'high' and subsequent crash, so avoid eating them.

Protein

Proteins are long chains of amino acids. Amino acids are the building blocks of proteins. The body can make some amino acids, but others must be obtained from food. Our bodies have over 100,000 different proteins with a vast array of essential functions. Proteins create DNA, synthesize muscle tissue, repair cells, digest food, and make new body parts when they wear out (yes, that happens). There are twenty amino acids, nine of which are termed "essential". The body cannot make the "essential" amino acids, so they must come from the food that you eat.

Many people incorrectly believe that protein only comes from animal flesh. Think about that for a second. If you eat a cow and the cow flesh has protein, but the cow didn't eat another cow to make that flesh, then where did the cow get her protein? From plants! All plant foods have protein—some more than others.

Protein-rich foods include vegetables such as broccoli (what??), beans, lentils, and whole grains. Nuts also have a lot of protein but contain a lot of fat, so eat nuts for their fatty acids, not their protein content.

Of all the plant foods, fruit has the least protein. It is still present, just in smaller quantities.

Fat

Your brain is comprised of about 60% fat. Fat is essential for your brain. But what about the rest of your body? Is fat good for your liver or your butt? Let's dive into that.

Most natural foods already have some fat in them, just as they contain protein and carbohydrates. Take broccoli, for example: it is 64% carbohydrates, 26% protein and 10% fat. Yep, even broccoli has protein and fat. Even lettuce, yes lettuce, contains about 4% fat. So all the fat you need could come from whole foods alone. Don't get me wrong; I'm not saying you should survive on a diet of broccoli and lettuce. However, what I am saying is that you don't need added fats in your diet to thrive.

Yes, bodies need fat for essential functions, but not the extra fat from oils or spreads. While nuts and seeds are healthy, they're also packed with fat, so eat them sparingly.

Whenever I talk to people about improving their health, the topic of olive oil always comes up. People have been led to believe it is a "healthy fat." Here's the deal: olive oil is primarily oleic acid, an omega-9 monounsaturated fat. While you need omega-9 fatty acids in small quantities, it's not essential, the body can make it's own from other fatty acids. Olive oil is slightly healthier than coconut oil, which is 80-90% saturated fat. Olive oil is a highly processed version of an olive. All the fiber and many nutrients are removed. Like other oils, it packs more calories per gram than anything else you eat — nine calories per gram, in fact.

Here's the bottom line: feast on a wide variety of whole plants. Want an olive? Go for it. Have a few (just don't eat the entire jar). When it comes to oil, say goodbye to it. Why? Because oil is high in calories with hardly any of the vitamins, fiber, or goodness that comes with whole foods. You could have an extra-large banana—filled with potassium, vitamin B6, vitamin C, fiber, and deliciousness—or a tablespoon of oil, which offers minimal nutritional value and heads straight for your love handles. Which sounds better? So, from now on, let's make oil a thing of the past. It's officially dead to you!

Micronutrients

I'm sure you can guess by the name micro that these guys are little. Micronutrients are the tiny molecules inside the macronutrients. Micronutrients comprise vitamins, minerals, and phytonutrients – tiny plant substances that pack a healthy power punch. You may have heard of words like polyphenols, flavanols, and antioxidants – these are all phytonutrients. Micronutrients are the workhorses of food. They act as catalysts to make reactions happen. You need them for all processes of bodily function. Without them, you are dead.

Many people who are overweight are eating a lot of food with very few micronutrients – think processed and fast food. It is entirely possible to be malnourished and still overweight. Read that again.

How does that happen?

When you eat processed and manufactured foods, you ingest many calories for energy. These are the macronutrients: protein, fat, and carbohydrates. However, if that food is nutrient-poor, your body will keep searching for micronutrients. When they are not found, your brain thinks you are still hungry. So, even though you are getting a lot of energy (calories), you are not getting enough nutrition (micronutrients). Your body wants nutrients, not excess calories. This is why you can still feel hungry after a big fast-food meal. Crazy, right?

Vitamins

There are two types of vitamins: water-soluble and fat-soluble. As the name suggests, water-soluble vitamins dissolve in water. People need to eat foods containing these vitamins every day. Fat-soluble vitamins dissolve in fat and can be stored in body fat.

The water-soluble vitamins are the B vitamins group (including folate) and vitamin C. Fat-soluble vitamins are vitamins A, D, E, and K. You can absorb more of these vitamins when you eat foods containing fat. For example, the vitamin A in tomatoes will be better absorbed when you eat them with avocado, which contains fat and vitamin E.

But don't stress. If you eat a whole plant foods diet, you won't need to combine food or calculate vitamin intake. People who don't eat many vegetables or fruit may be concerned about their vitamin intake, but not you. The human body is so amazing that it will take all the vitamins you eat, use what it needs, and discard the rest. So you don't need to eat tomato and avocado together to get the benefits. (You can, because it's yummy!) You will still be getting abundant nutrition without really trying.

Minerals

Minerals come from the earth. The ones used in our bodies include calcium, magnesium, potassium, sodium, iron, zinc, phosphorus, chloride, iodine and selenium. They have a wide range of functions and are required in varying amounts. Again, do not worry about learning the recommended daily allowance of dietary minerals unless you suspect a deficiency. However, if you were wondering, here's a non-exhaustive list of why you need these minerals.

- Calcium—bone health*, blood clotting, nerve transmission, muscle contraction.

*Women especially need to be aware of their calcium status. After menopause, bone density naturally decreases.

- Magnesium—muscle relaxation, DNA, bone and tissue formulation, regulation of blood sugar.
- Potassium—fluid and electrolyte regulation, maintains steady heartbeat, part of bone.
- Sodium—fluid regulation, nerve transmission, muscle contraction.
- Iron—growth and development, transportation of oxygen to red blood cells, hormones.
- Zinc—growth and development—fetal and during puberty, particularly for boys, wound healing, eye health, blood clotting.
- Phosphorus—ATP (adenosine triphosphate)—the body's energy currency, cell membranes, bones.
- Chloride—maintains fluid and electrolyte balance and synthesizes stomach acid.
- Iodine—production of thyroid hormones, growth, development, temperature regulation, nerve and muscle function.
- Selenium—production of thyroid hormones, works with vitamin E as an antioxidant, anticancer effects.

All these minerals can be found in a varied diet of whole plant foods.

Phytonutrients

The word phytonutrient means nourishment from plants. It's a general term because thousands of phytonutrients haven't been thoroughly investigated. Scientists estimate there are 25,000 different phytonutrients in plant foods [79]. Phytonutrients help prevent and potentially reverse many diseases, including cancer, cardiovascular disease, cognitive decline, and diabetes. There are different classes of phytonutrients: carotenoids, flavonoids, lignans, phenolic acids, polyphenols, sterols, and terpenes. These words may seem foreign to you, so let's talk briefly about some of them and how they affect our health.

Carotenoids are found in red and orange fruit and vegetables, including carrots, squash, citrus fruit, and mangoes. These are also antioxidants and can decrease the risk of cancer. Avoid carotenoid supplements. Only whole foods have these benefits.

Flavonoids can be broken down into many classes. Flavones are found in celery, red peppers, citrus, and mint. Flavonols are found in onions, tomatoes, lettuce, kale, apples, grapes, tea and berries. Isoflavonoids are found in soybeans and legumes [80]. Flavonoids have many functions in the human body most notably antioxidant and anti-inflammatory properties.

Anthocyanins are a subclass of flavonoids. They are easy to spot because they appear with dark blue or purple pigments in dark berries, beets, cabbage, and eggplant skin. These pigments have antioxidant capabilities, which means they stop cell oxidation and slow down cell aging. That is why berries are so good for a youthful appearance and slowing down age-related cognitive decline. Awesome, hey?

Lignans are mainly found in seeds, especially flax, which has up to 700 times more lignans than other plants. Other sources of lignans include nuts, beans, and soy. Fruit and vegetables also contain lignans with diverse potencies [81]. Recent research has suggested that lignans have antitumor, anti-estrogenic, anti-inflammatory, and antiviral properties [82]. Lignans act as phytoestrogens, which can lower the risk of heart disease, menopause symptoms, breast cancer, and osteoporosis [81].

Plant sterols get a lot of press for their cholesterol and triglyceride-lowering properties. Plant sterols slow down the process of atherosclerosis and, in turn, reduce the risk of heart disease [83]. However, you need about one gram of plant sterols daily to lower cholesterol. You must eat about two pounds (1kg) of whole grains or four pounds (2kg) of fruit and vegetables daily to get this many sterols. On a whole plant foods diet, it is possible to absorb this amount of sterols; however, if you have high cholesterol, do not self-treat solely with food. High cholesterol significantly raises the risk of heart attacks and strokes.

Adaptogens

What is an adaptogen? Sometimes the word adaptogen is a buzzword manufacturers like to add to their products, such as teas and protein powders. But do these foods have health properties? The Cleveland Clinic describes adaptogens as 'plants and mushrooms that help your body respond to stress, anxiety, fatigue, and overall wellbeing' [84]. Common adaptogens are ashwagandha, ginseng, and some mushrooms. Adaptogens may be beneficial or an expensive waste of money, depending upon their origin and dose. Avoid randomly buying buckets of them online. They may sound incredible, but there is potential for adverse reactions with certain medications. Remember—just because it's natural or a herb does not mean it is safe or beneficial for your health. I'm not saying that adaptogens are not safe; just check with your doctor first before adding them to your routine.

Antinutrients

Oh, antinutrients! "Don't eat spinach because it's full of oxalates!" "The phytic acid in grains will leach calcium from your bones!" Have you seen these claims on the internet and believed them? Whenever I read a headline claiming a particular plant food has 'antinutrients,' I have a little chuckle. What is the claimant selling? What benefits them by steering you away from spinach or grains? My guess is they are steering you toward their grain-free product, that's what.

Sure, some whole plant foods contain compounds called phytates that might make some minerals slightly less bioavailable. Overall, the benefits of eating a wide variety of whole plant foods with their extensive matrix of phytonutrients, fiber, vitamins, and minerals, far outweigh any absorption discrepancies. PLEASE! Ignore the naysayers who make these claims and continue to eat as wide a variety of plant foods as is available to you.

> I will mention a caveat here. If you are diagnosed as deficient in specific minerals, you may need to pay attention to phytic acid. Pickling, fermenting, sprouting, and cooking can reduce the amount of phytic acid in whole foods.

Supplements

Vitamins are only beneficial to the human body if they are deficient. Excess supplemental vitamins are, at best, a waste of money and, at worst, toxic. Please do not pop high-dose vitamins willy-nilly without determining your vitamin status. You will need a blood test to check this. Below are the vitamins and minerals you may wish to use to supplement your diet.

Vitamin B12

Vitamin B12 is a micronutrient not available within whole plant foods. Microbes within the soil synthesize it. Historically, vitamin B12 attached itself to root vegetables. Unfortunately, with soil nutrient depletion a worldwide concern, plant-based eaters can no longer rely on soil bacteria for their vitamin B12, so you MUST supplement. Yes, 'MUST' is in capital letters.

This is **NOT NEGOTIABLE**.

If you want to be alive, you need vitamin B12—only a teeny weeny amount, but you need it. The universally accepted recommended daily allowance (RDA) is 2.4 micrograms (μg). However, vitamin B12 supplementation is not readily bioavailable, so a 100μg supplement may only be about 2%

bioavailable. So, taking 100μg gives you around 2μg. I take 100 micrograms daily and eat vitamin B12-fortified foods to compensate for any shortfall.

Alternatively, you can take 1000-2500μg once per week. Some foods are fortified with vitamin B12, including nutritional yeast, breakfast cereals, tempeh, and soy milk. However, due to these products' varying amounts and inconsistent use, it is advised not to rely solely on them for your total vitamin B12 intake.

There are four types of vitamin B12. Two of them, methylcobalamin and cyanocobalamin, are manufactured as vitamin supplements. The methyl type is active, and the cyanotype is inactive, but the body converts it to the active form. The difference is that the methyl type has a methyl unit attached, and the cyano has a cyanide unit attached.

I prefer methylcobalamin over cyanocobalamin. More research has been done on cyanocobalamin because it's a lot cheaper. The general scientific consensus is that it really doesn't matter which type you use; just take it. Make sure to choose a respected brand of vitamins with a seal of authenticity. This is the verified mark of the United States Pharmacopeia (USP) in America. In Europe, vitamins and supplements are monitored by the European Food Safety Authority.

Vitamin D

Natural plant foods do not contain vitamin D, but some foods are fortified with this vitamin. Our bodies manufacture vitamin D from the sun's radiation. As many of us spend a lot of daylight hours inside, some people don't get enough sunlight to make adequate vitamin D. Additionally, the fear of skin cancer can keep us out of the sun and risk becoming vitamin D deficient.

Vitamin D is an essential micronutrient for the formation of bone cells. It works with calcium to make new bone cells and help prevent age-onset osteoporosis. Osteoporosis is the gradual degradation of our bone tissue, making our bones brittle and more prone to fracture.

Vitamin D is also essential for nerve and muscle function and boosting immunity to fight pathogens like bacteria and viruses.

Supplementing with vitamin D has also been shown to help lower blood pressure and reduce the risk of heart disease. It can also help regulate blood sugar and help the brain function properly [85].

Adults need about 600 IU (15 mg) per day. If you are a post-menopausal woman who takes calcium, check the label of your supplement, as it may also contain vitamin D.

There are two different types of vitamin D. Vitamin D2 (ergocalciferol) and vitamin D3 (cholecalciferol). I recommend supplementing with vitamin D3 as it is more effectively converted into it's active form in the body. Some vitamin D supplements are sourced from lanolin, an animal product. If you want a plant-based option, go for one sourced from lichen. The bottle should say 'vegan'.

Calcium

Calcium is used for building bones. It is also essential for heart health and can help keep blood pressure low. Calcium is abundant in almonds, sesame seeds, tofu, leafy greens, lentils, and fortified plant milks. Some greens, such as spinach and Swiss chard, contain oxalates that reduce calcium absorption. But don't stress; you can still eat those yummy foods for the other beneficial vitamins and minerals they contain.

You may have heard that plant calcium is less bioavailable than from dairy products. That is completely bogus. Kale contains five times more bioavailable calcium than skim milk [86].

There has been some discussion that high supplemental calcium can increase the risk of cardiovascular disease. Not all studies show this effect, and it depends on the amount of calcium taken and for how long. I take calcium as I believe the benefits outweigh the risks.

Omega 3

Omega-3 is the most essential fatty acid for human health. Omega-3 fatty acids are in the membrane of every cell in our body. Over a third of the fat in the brain is omega-3. Omega-3 fatty acids can reduce symptoms of depression and the risk of cardiovascular disease and cancer. They also help to reduce inflammation, so they are beneficial for people with metabolic syndrome and rheumatoid arthritis and to help prevent dementia.

Omega-3 fatty acids are not made by the body and must be obtained from the diet. Walnuts, flax, and chia seeds are the best food sources of omega-3 fatty acids. To obtain adequate omega-3 fatty acids, eat about 30gm (1 oz) of walnuts or a tablespoon of flax or chia seeds daily.

Many people associate omega-3 fatty acids with fish oil. Consider this: Many fish oil supplements can be rancid even before you open the bottle, and if they're not, they can be contaminated with mercury. So, for me, no thanks! Here's a little secret: fish get their omega-3s from algae. And guess what? So can we! Look for omega-3 supplements derived from algae or ahi flower extract. That's where the real, clean stuff is.

Vitamin C

Vitamin C is a powerful antioxidant and an important part of human metabolism. Vitamin C is water-soluble, so our bodies don't store a lot of it. This means you need to be eating adequate amounts of it daily. Adults need between 75—90 mg of vitamin C daily (more for pregnant women) [87]. This can be easily obtained with food. Eating food containing vitamin C enhances the absorption of iron in meals. Here are some examples of a food's vitamin C content for a 100gm serving:

Red bell pepper—142 mg

Kale—93 mg

Broccoli—91 mg

Kiwi fruit—59 mg

Strawberries—60 mg

Orange—59 mg

As you can see, there is no shortage of vitamin C in fresh fruit and vegetables.

Multivitamins

My clients often ask me if they should take a multivitamin. I do not recommend across-the-board supplementation. If you are eating enough high-quality whole food, you should be able to get most of your nutrients from your food. Sometimes, that is not the case, and the body does not process the nutrients as it should, so a little targeted help might be required. Nutritional supplements are generally not regulated by the Food and Drug Administration. The only thing they regulate is the label that can go on the bottle. They do not check if what is claimed on the label is true! If you buy a bottle of 300 multivitamin tablets for five dollars at the supermarket, you can almost guarantee you are purchasing a bottle of rubbish. Additionally, they may be harmful to you rather than helpful.

A multivitamin, even a high-quality one, may not give you the expected benefits. Excess vitamin A supplementation, for example, can be harmful, as can excess iron. It's best to focus on the essential supplements (vitamin B12) and ask your doctor to test you regularly for vitamin D status and discuss calcium and omega-3 with them.

Workbook

Quiz

1. Name the four macronutrients.

Answer True of False

2. Most foods have some proportion of the three main macronutrients.
3. Vitamins and minerals are found abundantly in olive oil.
4. All plants have protein, and a varied whole plant foods diet can supply me with all my protein needs.

ANSWERS in Appendix

Journal

Today I learned
___

Today I feel
___

I am proud of myself today because
___

One thing I can improve upon tomorrow is
___

What is my biggest struggle right now?
___

Who can I ask to support me with this?
___

What is my main goal this week?
___

What does my idea of success look like next week?
___
___
___
___

What three daily actions can I take to reach that goal?

1. _____

   _____

2. _____

   _____

3. _____

   _____

> **Quick Tip**
>
> It is easy to get bogged down in the science of nutrition. Rather than looking at individual nutrients, concentrate on eating a wide variety from all the food groups: vegetables, fruit, whole grains, legumes, nuts and seeds, and herbs and spices. If in doubt, check your levels before buying lots of random supplements.

CHAPTER 7: A New Way of Eating

"Let food be thy medicine, and medicine be thy food." Hippocrates

What's In This Chapter?

This chapter explains the acronym ASOUPAS and helps you identify ASOUPAS foods. Don't stress, I'll explain shortly. You will learn why these foods are detrimental to your health and what alternatives you can eat right now to benefit your health.

What Is ASOUPAS Free?

I coined an acronym: ASOUPAS. Other people use part of this acronym. You may have heard of S.O.S free. It stands for free from sugar, oil, and salt. It's popular amongst many plant-based eaters. But I'm taking it a few steps further because I want you to succeed immediately. Dr. Dean Ornish, one of the most eminent scientists in the world of lifestyle disease reversal, says that moderation sometimes is not enough to elicit meaningful change and intensive intervention will get you the results you crave. (I'm paraphrasing). So go all in. I want you to thrive and be as healthy as possible.

ASOUPAS stands for Animal products, Sugar, Oil, Ultra-Processed foods, Alcohol, and Salt.

ASOUPAS are not beneficial for your long-term health.

These six foods are also the culprits that stop you from losing weight. This might not be too much of a change for some of you already on a plant-based diet. You are already halfway there. However, if you are currently eating the Standard American/Australian diet (the acronym for that diet is aptly, S.A.D), this could seem like a mountain too big to climb. Fear not. I know you can climb it, and I know you will climb it – and it won't be half as difficult as you imagine. In fact, it's going to be delicious.

Let's look at these foods individually and why you want to remove them from your diet.

Animal Products

If you think right now there is no way you can possibly give up your hamburger and still be alive, stay tuned. I have some tricks up my sleeve that will allow you to have delicious and healthy burgers. The only difference is that they are made from plants, not animal flesh. Animal products contain saturated fat, hormones, chemicals, and veterinary medicines. Animal products are responsible for the obesity epidemic, diabetes, heart disease, and death! Get them out of your life immediately!

Sugar

When you eat carbohydrates, your body breaks them down to sugars, including glucose. Try to think of the words sugar and glucose as interchangeable. The body loves glucose; it is its preferred fuel source. Remember the engine room from Chapter 4? If you have forgotten how the body uses glucose, head back to Chapter 4 for a refresher.

In a perfect world, your body runs seamlessly on glucose, but that doesn't mean you should add sugar to your diet. There is enough glucose in natural fruit, whole grains, and vegetables to satisfy the body's metabolic needs. Added sugar is detrimental to our bodies and harmful to weight loss. If the extra calories in your diet come from sugar, the body will convert them to fat and store them as love handles. The sad part is sugar is in everything! Pickles, tomato sauce, peanut butter. Foods that don't need sugar in them now have it.

But what is worse than sugar? High fructose corn syrup. This ubiquitous fake food has infiltrated the food system, so it's tough to avoid it if you buy ultra-processed foods. The other day, I saw a soda can with the health claim, "Now with real sugar!" As if that's a bonus! High fructose corn syrup is a major player in the incidence of diabetes, some cancers, non-alcoholic fatty liver disease, and cardiovascular and kidney diseases [88]. It is banned in many countries, yet accounts for 40% of added sweetener in the American diet. This is madness!

When I urge you to avoid added sugar, I do not mean for you to avoid fruit. Please avoid processed foods with added sugars, such as cakes, desserts, candy, fizzy drinks (sodas), juices, breakfast cereals, ready meals, and fast food.

Sugar can be sneaked into processed foods under many names. Always read food labels (more in Chapter 12) and avoid all the following: sugar, high fructose corn syrup, agave nectar, brown rice syrup, coconut sugar, evaporated cane juice, fruit juice concentrate, turbinado sugar, molasses, dextrose, maltose, honey, crystalline fructose and anything that ends in the word syrup.

Oil

Oil is highly processed and has nine calories per gram. It's the most energy-dense food available. If weight loss is your goal, then banish oil from your kitchen. Despite the claims from oil lovers, oil is not full of antioxidants and nutrients. Olives are chock full of health-promoting phytochemicals, but the oil, sadly, is primarily bereft of them. All that lovely fiber and phytonutrients have been left behind in the extraction process.

Additionally, olive oil can contain up to 20% palmitic acid, a saturated fat. Palmitic acid increases inflammation that can lead to an added risk of atherosclerosis and cardiovascular diseases [89, 90]. To maintain health, you need to reduce your saturated fat content. The American Heart Association recommends a diet containing no more than 6% saturated fat. You will only achieve that goal if you ditch the oil.

If that's not enough to sway you, consider this. A tablespoon of oil has 135 calories in the USA and 180 calories in Australia (because tablespoons are larger in Australia). Even if all you did to change your diet was reduce oil by one tablespoon daily, you would save between 49,000 and 66,000 calories annually. This theoretically equates to a weight loss between 14 and 18 pounds (6-8 kg)!

Now, think about those corn chips at the Mexican restaurant. Those fries with your burger. That donut at morning tea. They are all fried in oil. Imagine how many calories you will save by eliminating the oil. Remember this—if you are overweight or obese, weight loss leads to better health and less disease risk. You can still have corn chips, fries, and donuts—you just need to be in control of their cooking processes.

Before you throw this book in the trash for my anti-oil heresy, I have solutions to your oily desires. Think about what you use oil for. Is it to stop food sticking to the bottom of the pan? To make the food brown? To make food taste better?

If you use oil so food doesn't stick to your pan, try a non-stick pan such as enamel or cast iron. For fat-free stir-frying, try salt-free vegetable stock or water. Use an air fryer or hot oven for crispy fries and potato chips. Yum. Oil coats your taste buds and hides the flavor of the food. Once you start using oil-free cooking methods, you will wonder why you ever used oil in the first place.

Ultra-Processed Foods

Food processing is classified according to the NOVA scale. NOVA ranks foods from least processed to most processed. For example, Group 1 includes unprocessed or minimally processed foods, including fresh or frozen fruit and vegetables, whole grains, and legumes. Group 4 includes ultra-processed food and drink products, including highly processed industrial foods with many ingredients not limited to food, such as dyes, isolates, flavor enhancers, and other chemicals [91].

Have you ever picked up some tortillas and expected the ingredients to be corn, water, and maybe some salt? Only to find the ingredients are corn masa flour, interesterified and hydrogenated soybean oils, salt, water, cellulose gum, guar gum, propionic acid, amylase, benzoic acid, and phosphoric acid. What? Yes, some of those ingredients are preservatives, so they don't go moldy as soon as you get them home. What about the rest? Are they really needed? Remember when bread went moldy after three days? That's because it was made with real ingredients.

The issue with ultra-processed foods is that many are not 'food' at all. They are food-like products masquerading as food. They have flavor enhancers, artificial sweeteners, gums, modified starches, and chemicals that humans should never ingest.

Take titanium dioxide, for example. This is an ingredient in sunscreen and ice cream! Hello! Why is there sunscreen in my ice cream? Because it makes the ice cream, frosting, or candy light and bright. Titanium dioxide (otherwise known as color E171) is banned in the European Union due to its connection to cancer [92]. But in the USA, it's everywhere. The FDA does not even require it to be listed as an ingredient. Food manufacturers can call it 'coloring.'

Ultra-processed foods are a convenience. They are not healthy. They will not help you regain your health. To stay healthy, stay away from ultra-processed food. Eat more Group 1 food and less Group 4 Frankenfoods.

Alcohol

I hope it is obvious why alcohol is off the list. First, alcohol impedes your judgment, so you are more likely to overeat. (Ooh, look! Cookies!) Second, alcohol is a depressant and a toxin. Alcohol is detrimental to brain health and has been implicated in the progression of dementia [13]. My favorite study on the effects of alcohol followed 500 people for thirty years and compared the amount of alcohol they drank with how well their brains worked. Even moderate drinkers showed brain damage and shrinkage [93]! So, get alcohol out of your life.

I recently recorded a podcast on this very subject. Check out The Fabulous Health Show and look at episode 24, *How Much Alcohol is Too Much?* You can also watch it on my YouTube channel, Fabulous Health.

Third, alcohol has seven calories per gram, and the body burns it preferentially over other macronutrients. Why? Because it is poison, and the body wants to use it as fast as possible. What does burning alcohol preferentially mean? If you have an alcoholic drink and a piece of cake, your body will use the alcohol as energy and slap that piece of cake right on your butt in your fat cells. No thanks.

I get it. Here I am on my high horse telling you to ditch the booze. It might be hard for you. Wine might be part of your culture. Your social life might revolve around alcohol.

Let's say you like the social connection alcohol brings, and you have wine with dinner and a few drinks on the weekends. Try weaning yourself from it gradually. Make every second drink a non-alcoholic one and reduce from there. You don't have to tell the world; just order a soda water with lime and move on. It's none of anyone else's business anyway. If someone is pressuring you to drink alcohol, it might be time to re-evaluate your relationship with that person.

When you know that alcohol is harmful to your mind and body, there's a choice you have to make. Ditch it or suffer the consequences.

> **IMPORTANT:** If you feel that giving up alcohol would be extremely difficult, you may have an addiction. Please seek professional advice from a qualified addiction counselor. Check the resources for more information.

Salt

Natural foods have enough sodium for our bodies to function optimally. Excess sodium can lead to hypertension (high blood pressure) and increase your risk of heart disease, stroke, osteoporosis, kidney disease, and cancer. Salt also loves water. Where there is salt, water follows. So, if you don't want to be bloated all the time, ditch the salt.

Natural plant foods do not contain sodium in amounts you should be concerned about. If you are confused about the amount of sodium in a packaged food, look at the label. If the amount of sodium in a serving is about the same as the number of calories, then the product has an acceptable amount of sodium. If not, put that product back on the supermarket shelf.

See the illustration on the next page. the product has 2.3 times the healthy amount of sodium. Once you start reading labels, you will be shocked at the amount of sodium in packaged foods.

Nutrition Facts	
Serving Size: 1 ounce (28.35g)	
Calories 100 % Daily Value*	
Amount per serving	
Total Fat 10g	15%
Saturated Fat 5g	25%
Trans Fat 0g	0%
Cholesterol 30mg	10%
Sodium 230mg	10%
Total Carbohydrate 0g	0%
Dietary Fiber 0g	0%
Total sugars 0g	
Added sugars 0g	0%
Protein 7g	14%

*The % daily value tells you how much a nutrient in a serving of food contributes to a daily diet. 2000 calories a day is used for general nutrition advice

---

When you stop cooking with salt and eating packaged foods with added sodium, you may see a quick drop in weight and blood pressure. If you are on blood pressure meds, please monitor your blood pressure daily.

The World Health Organization recommends eating a maximum of 2000mg of sodium daily [94]. That's about one teaspoon of table salt. Before you ask, that includes Himalayan pink salt, Celtic sea salt, and Kosher salt. If you add salt to your food, please use iodized salt and do so at the table. Iodized salt contains trace amounts of iodine, an essential nutrient. Your taste buds will taste the salt on top of your food. If you add salt to cooking, it will disperse, and you can potentially add too much. Alternatively, try kelp granules. They taste salty and are a great source of iodine, but contain no sodium. Win-win!

Workbook

Quiz

1. What does ASOUPAS stand for?
2. Fill in the blank. Oil has ..... calories per gram, and alcohol has ..... calories per gram.

Answer True or False

3. This book focuses on eating more ASOUPAS foods.
4. Even though the body runs on sugar (glucose), excess sugar is dangerous .
5. White flour has most of its fiber removed.
6. Whole plant foods already contain enough sodium for the human body.

ANSWERS in Appendix

Journal

Today I learned
_____

Today I feel
_____

I am proud of myself today because
_____

One thing I can improve upon tomorrow is
_____

What is my biggest struggle right now?
_____

Who can I ask to support me with this?
_____

What is my main goal this week?
_____

What does my idea of success look like next week?
_____
_____
_____

What three daily actions can I take to reach that goal?

1. _____

   _____

2. _____

   _____

3. _____

   _____

> **Quick Tip**
>
> Instead of focusing on what you leave off your plate, focus on the infinite array of delicious, whole foods you will add to your meals. If you are overwhelmed already, just relax. Breathe in, breathe out. Think about how amazing you will feel when you remove poisons from your body and start fueling it with delicious, nutritious food. I've already mentioned that you will get the quickest results if you go all in. But if that is too much, and you are not suffering from a life-threatening condition such as advanced heart disease, then take it slow. Go at your own pace. It's your life. Make the most effortless changes first and progress from there. I'll talk more about that in Chapter 10. Stay with me.

CHAPTER 8: Setting Up For Success

"He who is not courageous enough to take risks will accomplish nothing in life." Muhammad Ali

What's In This Chapter?

This chapter is your starting point for real change. You will take starting measurements of all your health parameters. You may be loathe to take measurements at the start of your journey, but later, you will be glad you did. Don't be scared. It's just data.

Know Your Numbers

How will you know you have succeeded if you don't measure your progress? Measurement is imperative if you want to see and understand change. Sometimes, you might look in the mirror and think there has been no change. Or you jump on the scale, and the number goes up instead of down. Then, you get discouraged and are more likely to give up.

So many things are happening in your body when you start to improve your health. There are things you can't see, like improved glucose control, lower blood pressure, and improved liver function. These biometric measurements are far more critical than the number on a scale, and they give you a better indication of your health than your pants size.

So, before you do anything. **KNOW YOUR NUMBERS.**

Blood Tests

Make an appointment with your doctor and ask for a full blood panel. Sometimes, this is called a *well person* blood panel. If you live in the USA, your insurance often covers this annually. You will want to measure at least the following biometric parameters:

Total Cholesterol

LDL Cholesterol (bonus points for measuring ApoB)

HDL Cholesterol

Triglycerides

HbA1c

Liver Panel

Thyroid Panel

Serum Vitamin B12 (bonus points for measuring Homocysteine)

Serum Vitamin D

C-Reactive Protein

Blood Pressure (sphygmomanometer)

Fasting Glucose (urine test)

Once you have taken these tests and you have permission from your doctor to change your diet, you are good to go. These tests may reveal things you didn't want to know. You may be worried that some measurements are high or abnormal. Don't stress. You are about to change all that.

> IMPORTANT: Once you start fueling your body with nutrients and stop assaulting it with toxins, your body may begin to heal itself. Over time, you may need less medication, so keep in close contact with your doctor and consult them if you have any concerns. Do not stop taking any medications without express permission from your primary care provider.

Body Measurements

Aaaaagh! "You want me to take measurements and pictures? No way, Jose!"

Stop right there. Listen to yourself. Why don't you want to take measurements and pictures? Is it because you are embarrassed? Or do you not want to know the truth? Own who you are right now. No blame. No pretense. You are as you are, and you are a beautiful person. You may not be as healthy as you wish, and you may be carrying extra pounds – but that will change starting right now.

Why do I make you do this? So that you can look back in a few months and be amazed at how far you have come. So you can be proud of the effort you put in and the progress you have made. No one has to see these photos. No one has to know your measurements. They are only for you. So, suck it up, Princess. Do the dang photos and the measurements and move on.

Weight

Wake up, go to the toilet, strip naked, and weigh yourself. Just for fun, do this for five days in a row and notice the changes. Are you the same weight every day? I bet not. This is proof that your body weight changes daily and is not a reliable measurement of health. Don't get hung up on the scale. Some days, it will be your friend, other days, not so much. Weigh yourself, write it down, and forget about it.

> Always use the same scale at the same time of day, naked if possible. Then, you can compare measurements accurately. Don't be discouraged when you weigh more when you're fully clothed at the doctor's office.

Height

You will need help with this. I know you think you are 5'8", but when they measure you at the doctor's office, you are only 5'6". Guess what? You are 5'6". If you can't get professionally measured, get a family member to help you at home.

Take your shoes off and stand with your heels and back against a wall. Have someone taller than you place a set square (triangle ruler) against the wall with the right angle on top of your head.

Take a deep breath and lower your shoulders. With the back of your head against the wall, drop your chin a little and look down toward the ground about a meter (3 feet) ahead of you. Mark the wall under the set square. If you want, do it three times and take the average. If your measuring helper measures correctly, all three measurements should be the same.

Anthropometric and Biometric Measurements

Anthropometric measurement is just a fancy word for measuring the circumference of your limbs with a tape measure. Biometric measurements measure your body fat percentage. Both are helpful measurements, but, like all measurements, some are more prone to error than others. Some of these measurements are essential, and others are optional. However, you need to complete at least one of these options.

1. Gold Standard – DEXA

DEXA stands for Dual Energy X-ray Absorptiometry and is the gold standard of body composition. As expected, it is also the most expensive way of determining how much fat and muscle you have in your body. Some insurance providers may sponsor part of a DEXA scan, but others may not. Please check if this is available to you. I got one for $79 USD on Groupon without using my health insurance.

DEXA also measures bone density; if you are a woman, it's good to know if you are at risk of osteoporosis. DEXA uses two x-rays to measure both soft tissue and bone tissue. It is also the only device that measures visceral fat (the fat surrounding your internal organs) and is a good indicator of disease risk.

For more information on DEXA, watch this video from the manufacturer General Electric on their YouTube channel GE HealthCare.

youtu.be/Y7aum8ry3y4

For details about the scan and report, watch this video from the Utah State University Extension.

youtu.be/tZZol83tv14

Have a DEXA scan now and then again in six or twelve months. It's not practical to do a DEXA every week or every month. Don't stress about the radiation, as DEXA emits much less radiation than a chest x-ray. I recommend getting at least one DEXA scan if you can afford it.

2. Bioimpedance

You may have a body fat analysis scale at home or in your gym. These work via bioimpedance. An electrical current travels through your body, and the scale determines how much fat you have based on the time it takes the current to return to the scale. Fat has a density different from muscle and other tissue, so the current travels at a speed different from that of other tissues. These machines are notoriously inaccurate, and results can change depending on your hydration levels. I urge you not to rely on them. If you have a body fat scale at home, please use it only to weigh yourself and don't heed the body fat calculation. It usually overestimates anyway, which is not good for your emotional well-being. You do not need to be told by a machine that you are fatter than you are.

If you go to an exercise physiology lab at a university, their bioimpedance machines are more accurate. Some universities use a machine called a BOD POD. Sometimes, students need test subjects, so contact your local sport and exercise department to see if you can get a BOD POD measurement. It's usually free.

Home Measurement of Body Fat

3. Navy Method

This is my favorite way of measuring body composition. It's cheap, accurate enough for our purposes, and easy to do. Irrespective of the more expensive methods, I advise you to measure your progress weekly using this method. You will need a regular dressmaker's tape measure (not a steel carpenter's tape), and you will measure:

- Your neck at the smallest part

- Your waist at the smallest part. If you do not have a visible waist, measure

1-2 inches (2-5 cm) above your belly button.

- Your hips at the widest part. This is usually around your pubis and the widest part of your butt cheeks. This measurement is required for females only.
- Your height.
- Your weight.

Watch this video to see how to do it.

youtube.com/watch?v=zW_sMFSzyy4&t=42s

The link above is the official US Navy video. The video uses a special tape measure, but you can use a normal one.

Enter your measurements here:

Tip: Use a pencil to rub them out and rewrite them later.

Neck: _____

Waist: _____

Hips: _____

Height: _____

Weight: _____

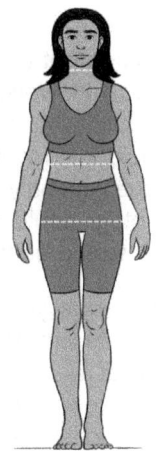
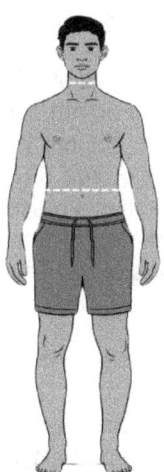

Body Fat Calculation

Then, plug the results into this calculator:

https://fabuloushealth.net/body-fat-calculator

This is the most important measurement you will make. When your body fat percentage decreases, the risk of diseases such as heart disease and diabetes also decreases.

If you are a science geek like me and want to know the math of the body fat calculator, you can use the formulas on the next page.

Body fat percentage (BFP) formula for females:

BFP = 163.205×log10 (waist + hip−neck)−97.684×(log10(height)) -78.387.

The optimal body fat percentage for females is 20-30%.

Body Fat Percentage (BFP) formula for males:

BFP = 86.010 x log10 (waist−neck)−70.041 x (log10 (height)) + 36.76.

Note that for men, the hip measurement is not used. The optimal body fat for males is 12-20%.

You can use the Navy method weekly to track your progress over time on a spreadsheet. Head to fabuloushealthbook.net/bonuses to enter your measurements. The spreadsheet will work its magic, so you don't need to remember the equation.

Other Measurements

1. The Scale

The scale is an obvious measurement choice for you if you are overweight and you do not currently exercise. However, it does not tell the entire picture. It does not tell you how much of you is water, bone, muscle, or fat. For example, two 5'8" people could both weigh 160 pounds. The first person could have a muscular physique with only 20% body fat (meaning they carry 32 pounds of fat), while the other could have 40% body fat and carry 64 pounds of fat. The first person would be much healthier than the second.

Many different things happen inside your body when you start improving your health. Health improvements are not necessarily reflected in a scale measurement. The scale does not measure your adherence to healthy habits or your blood pressure. The scale does not measure your hydration status or your sleep quality. If you are eating whole plant foods and the scale number is not budging, it might make you despondent and believe the program is not working. I can guarantee if you are following the program, good things are happening, and it is working!

Your weight loss will not be uniform. It may stall and sometimes your weight might go up a bit, but great things are happening inside you regardless of what the scale says. Use this tool as one of the measurement metrics in your arsenal, but please don't use it as the only measuring device.

2. Waist Measurement and Waist-to-Hip Ratio

Your waist-to-hip ratio is a good indicator of cardiovascular risk. A waist measurement of over 80cm (31.25in) for women and 94cm (37in) for men is associated with an increased risk of chronic diseases [95]. The ratio between your hip measurement and your waist measurement is also important. People who hold more fat in their mid-section (visceral fat) are more at risk of lifestyle diseases such as heart disease and diabetes than those who hold fat on their hips (subcutaneous fat). The optimal waist-to-hip ratio for a woman is 0.7 with disease risk increasing substantially once it reaches 0.85 (or 0.9 for men).

What do I mean by that? Let's say your waist is 70cm (27.5in) and your hips are 100cm (39in). Your waist-to-hip ratio is 70/100 = 0.7 (27.5/39 = 0.7) That's perfect! But what if your waist is 90cm (35.4in) and your hips are 100cm (39in)? Then your waist-to-hip ratio is 0.9, which is not so good.

A 2024 study from the UK showed that an increase in the waist-to-hip ratio is a predictor of cardiovascular disease, heart attack (especially for women), and stroke, independent of body fat percentage [95]. Regardless of your waist-to-hip ratio today, if you can bring it closer to 0.7 each week, you know you are on the right track.

What is my waist-to-hip ratio today?

_____

What starting method of body composition will I use to track my progress?

_____

_____

Starting Photos

Wait! Before you go running away in horror, hear me out. What if, in six months, when you are healthier and more gorgeous than you already are now, you want to look back at how far you have come? Wouldn't you want to celebrate that? I know I would.

You do not have to show me (or anyone) your 'before' photos. They are just for you. But please take them – for your own benefit.

Here's how you do it. You will need three photos.

Tips for great photos.

1. Have great lighting – a bathroom is usually good
2. Remove any background items such as kids' toys, dirty washing, etc. I usually take mine using a blank wall or a closed door as a background.

3. Wear athletic clothing such as a sports bra, shorts, or leggings and a fitted tank. The fewer clothes you wear, the better, but not too racy if you want to show others.

4. Get your whole body in the picture from top to toe. You can always crop later.

5. Most phones have a timer function so you can take the photos yourself.

6. When you do the repeat photos a few weeks later, make sure you are in the exact location, with the same lighting, and wearing the same clothing.

Go on. Get those photos done. File them away or show your friends and family. Whatever works for you. Just get them done.

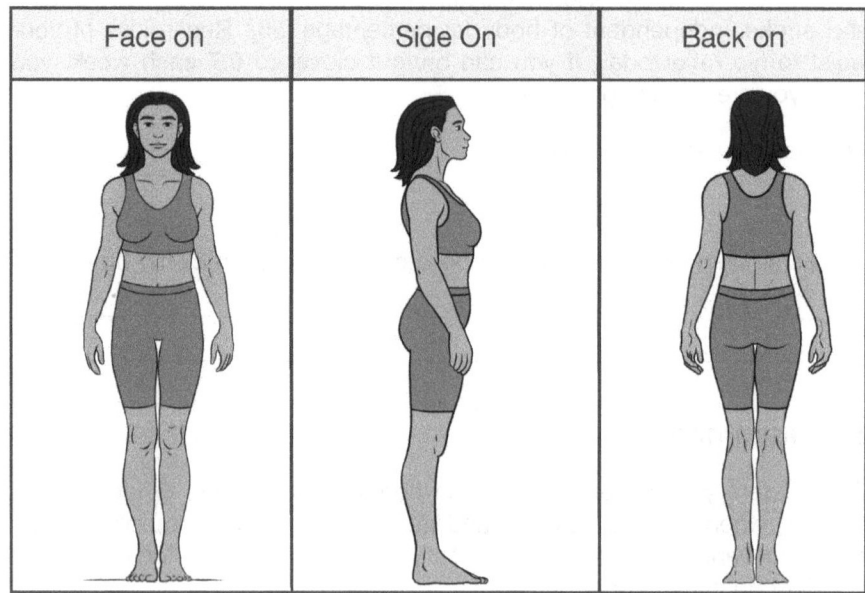

| Face on | Side On | Back on |

Goal Setting

Benjamin Franklin is famously quoted as saying, *"When you fail to plan, you plan to fail."* This is so true. Have you been winging your health journey up till now? How's that working out for you?

SMART Goals

Having goals is smart, but what are SMART goals? SMART stands for

Specific

Measurable

Attainable

Relevant

Time-bound

Do you want to lose weight? Get off your meds? Those are great goals, but they are not SMART goals. How much weight do you want to lose? How are you going to measure the weight loss? Is this a realistic amount of weight to lose? Can you achieve it in your current situation? How long will it take you to lose this amount of weight?

For all goals, make them SMART—not just in your head. Write them down. Nothing is set in concrete. You can always revisit them later and adapt them as necessary.

Here's an example:

I want to lose 20 pounds of fat over 20 weeks before my daughter's wedding. I will do so by eating a whole plant foods diet and exercising three times per week for one hour. I will shop weekly at the farmers market and prepare healthy meals. I will use the Navy method to measure my progress.

Specific: Lose 20 pounds for daughter's wedding

Measurable: Navy method

Attainable: 20 pounds in twenty weeks is attainable and a healthy time frame

Relevant: Yes, I want to look and feel my best. This aligns with my values.

Time-bound: Twenty weeks for daughter's wedding

This goal is specific, measurable, attainable, relevant, and time-bound. PERFECT!

Pick your top three SMART goals and fill in the information below. Don't stress if you only have one. One is better than none.

SMART GOAL No.1

S _____

M _____

A _____

R _____

T _____

Write your goal as an affirmation.

_____

_____

_____

_____

SMART GOAL No.2

S _____

M _____

A _____

R _____

T _____

Write your goal as an affirmation.

_____

_____

_____

_____

SMART GOAL No.3

S _____

M _____

A _____

R _____

T _____

Write your goal as an affirmation.

_____
_____
_____
_____
_____

It's Not All About Weight Loss

As I discussed in Chapter 4, most people looking to improve their health also want to lose weight. Excess fat is a risk factor for many other metabolic conditions. But don't get hung up on weight loss. Yes, losing weight can help lower your blood pressure, decrease joint pain, reduce your HbA1c (a measure of diabetes risk), and let you wear your skinny jeans. Weight loss is just one of many changes your body goes through on its way to optimal health. It is the most obvious because you can see it happening. What you can't see happening is lowering your inflammation, improving your hormone responses, and reducing the plaque in your arteries. All these magical things might be happening without you being aware of them.

You can't see these things happening, but you can feel them. Do you have more energy? Can you walk up the stairs without getting puffed? Can you do a squat without your knees burning? Are you sleeping better? Are your bowel movements more regular and less painful? All these data points are important and relevant and indicate that you are on the right track even if the scale or your skinny jeans trick you into believing they are not, so I urge you to keep a journal.

Keep A Journal

I'll be 100% transparent here. I love journals and planners. I have dozens of them; the first five pages are complete, and the rest are blank. I get all excited and then lose interest. That is because I start them without a clear reason to journal. As I write this book, I'm stuck on the couch, fresh from knee reconstruction surgery deemed necessary after a spill during the last ski season. Now, I have a reason to journal. I'm filling in that rehab journal every day. My exercises, pain medications, and how I'm feeling. Because I have a goal. A goal to progress from the brace and crutches and start walking. Then, a goal to get my knee to pre-injury strength so I can play tennis and go skiing again. When you have a big enough reason, you will follow through.

I can see some of you are ready to skip to the next chapter. You may not be a writer, and this disinterests you. That is fine, but please take notes on your phone, in an app, or in this book to see how you are progressing daily. You can record voice notes if writing is not your thing. There will be times when you think you are not making progress, and you will be tempted to give up and go back to old habits. I promise, if you do that, you will regret it. Use this book and just fill in the blanks. Get a calendar and scribble little milestones on it as they happen. Seeing how far you have come will give you a sense of pride and help you stay motivated to keep going.

Tracking Progress

It's up to you how you track your progress. There is only one rule. Be consistent! Weigh yourself on the same scale in the morning each week. Use the same tape measure, the same pair of pants, and the same walking route. Compare how you did today with how you did yesterday. If you get puffed walking around the block, note the day you didn't, or that you walked further than the day before. Your progress may not be linear. Scrub that. Your progress won't be linear. Sometimes, you'll progress; at other times, you will feel like you are going backward. Don't stress; this is normal. Just log it, move on, and watch the pattern.

Workbook

Quiz

1. What is considered the 'gold standard' of body composition measurement?
2. What is the optimal waist-to-hip ratio?

Answer True or False.

3. When measuring my body, I measure around my clothes.
4. There is no relationship between my waist measurement and my risk of lifestyle disease.
5. I can measure myself easily with the Navy Method.
6. I can wear anything I want for my 'before' photos.

ANSWERS in Appendix

Journal

Today I learned
_____
Today I feel
_____
I am proud of myself today because
_____
One thing I can improve upon tomorrow is
_____
What is my biggest struggle right now?
_____
Who can I ask to support me with this?
_____
What does my idea of success look like next week?
_____
_____
What is my main goal this week?
_____

What three daily actions can I take to reach that goal?

1._____

_____

2._____

_____

3._____

_____

Quick Tip

The more you monitor your progress, the more data points you will collect, and the better you will be at sticking to the program. Celebrate small and large wins, even if it's walking two blocks instead of one or choosing a fruit salad over a cupcake. Every decision can bring you closer to your goal. Read your journal often to remind yourself how awesome you are!

CHAPTER 9: Changing Your Environment

"The secret to longevity, as I see it, has less to do with diet, or even exercise, and more to do with the environment in which a person lives."
Dan Buettner, The Blue Zones

What's In This Chapter?

In this chapter, you will manipulate your environment, so your first choice is always healthy. You will learn how to say goodbye to the foods that no longer serve you and surround yourself with healthy options. You will also learn strategies to avoid the call of fast-food establishments.

Clean Out The Junk

For some of you, this chapter will be a piece of cake; for others, it will be the hardest thing to accomplish. Your environment is crucial to your success. If your kitchen is filled with unhealthy food, it will be harder for you to improve your health.

Cheese, chocolate, and anything processed with salt, sugar, and fat are as addictive as drugs. Eating them releases the neurotransmitter dopamine in the brain, making it difficult to stop eating [96]. These foods need to be removed from your environment. Think of them as your 'crack'. If a loved one was a crack addict, would you allow crack in your house? Hopefully not.

You might think you have the willpower of an ox and can keep unhealthy food in your house. Be aware that if food is in your home, you will eventually eat it. It might not be today, but you will eat it. The best thing for your sanity and success is to remove unhealthy foods from your environment. What do I mean by unhealthy foods?

- Meat, fish, poultry, game, deli meats, and all packaged foods containing animal products
- Dairy—milk, cheese, yogurt, ice cream, frozen desserts, and all packaged foods containing dairy
- Oil (you may keep an oil spray)
- Processed foods—breakfast cereals with added sugar, cake mixes, cookies, convenience foods, cup noodles
- Candy, chocolate, and snack foods

- TV dinners, frozen pizza
- Potato chips, corn chips, pretzels
- Salted and candied nuts
- Sodas and sugar sweetened beverages

You may be loath to throw away food. Or, maybe you can't afford to throw away food. Consider a food swap with your friends and family. Tell them you are trying to eat healthier and ask if they would like to swap (insert your poison) for some fresh produce from their garden or some fruit. It doesn't have to be an even swap. Give them everything.

Why would you want to poison your friends and family with the food that is making you sick? I know this sounds ridiculous. I could not give anyone I cared about food that contributes to disease. In my home, it would be in the trash. Choose your people wisely. Many people are uninterested in eating healthier and would happily accept your castaways.

Empty The Cabinets

My home is my haven. I spend more time there than anywhere else. I like to have my kitchen fully stocked with yummy food at all times so I can easily whip up a delicious meal or grab a quick snack. If my kitchen was filled with ice cream, potato chips, cookies, and cupcakes, I would eat them until they were gone. Then, I'd probably go to the supermarket and buy more.

This is why it is so important for our homes to be stocked only with healthy food, not food that contributes to weight gain and metabolic disease. If corn chips are in the cupboard, corn chips will be the snack of choice. However, if there are apples and bananas, fruit will be the snack of choice. I'm not saying you can never have another corn chip; you can make your own, and I'll show you how in Chapter 10. I'm trying to make it easier for you to choose healthier food. If your food environment is clean, you will eat clean.

Do an audit of your pantry, fridge and freezer and either donate unopened foods to a neighbor or friend or throw them out. Then, preferably right afterward, go shopping and fill your home with healthy, delicious food. Head to Chapter 10 to see what's on the menu. I have provided a handy shopping list to help you out.

The Easy Drive-through

We've all been there. You've had a busy day, it's late, you are hungry. Bam! Before you know it, you are in the drive-through getting a burger, fries, and a large soda. Then that 2000 calories of fried, processed junk is in your stomach. And you feel lousy. Why does this keep happening? Because it's a habit. I'll talk about making new habits in Chapter 20. But for now, I'll help you break the unconscious fast food consumption habit.

The easiest way to avoid buying fast food is to make it challenging to obtain. Take a different route home. It is almost impossible, in the USA at least, to drive more than 30 seconds without passing a fast food outlet. You probably have your favorite, and it is probably on the way home. Take the back roads. Avoid the temptation. If there was a vegan donut shop on my way home, I could not resist. Help yourself by making it more challenging to get take-out rubbish food than it is to go home and make healthy food. Even reheated leftover healthy food is better than drive-through 'frankenfood'.

Living With Others

What if other people in your home are not following your new healthy lifestyle? How can you ensure that you stay true to your health goals when family members or loved ones you live with don't want to eat the food you're eating?

My best advice is not to be confrontational about it. You do you, and let them do whatever makes them happy. If you are the main cook in your home, you could cook family-friendly plant-based meals, and if others want something non-compliant, they can fix it themselves.

As for all the non-compliant foods that others eat, ask that they be removed from the home or hidden somewhere you cannot access them. This is imperative. The only way to stay away from these foods is not to have them front and center. When you are hungry, you need healthy options close at hand. If other people insist on bringing unhealthy food into your home, gently ask them to keep their food out of the kitchen and in the garage or somewhere you will not see it.

Of course, if someone in your home loves oysters and you dislike oysters, there will be no temptation to eat them. The foods you know are triggers for you must be hidden.

Sodas And Sugar-Sweetened Beverages (SSBs)

Australians call them fizzy drinks; in America, they are called sodas. Researchers call them sugar-sweetened beverages (SSBs), and they include soda, fruit drinks, sports and energy drinks [97].

Irrespective of what you call them, these drinks are a significant source of excess sugar calories and a contributor to obesity. Studies also show that drinking SSBs has been associated with elevated triglycerides, cardiovascular disease, fatty liver disease, gout, and tooth cavities [98].

Do you want to know how much weight you can gain by drinking soda or sugary drinks?

Just one 20 ounce (600ml) bottle of regular soda has 270 calories. How many of those calories are from sugar? Go on, have a guess. ALL OF THEM! One hundred percent of the calories in a bottle of soda are from sugar! If you drink just one large soda per day, you take in 72 grams of added sugar daily. Over a year, this adds up to 26,280 grams (26.28 kilograms) or 58 pounds of sugar! Fifty-eight pounds of sugar has 105,120 calories. When you take in more calories than you burn, those excess calories are stored as fat. Those 105,120 calories equate to 30 pounds of excess fat. I'm not kidding! The math does not lie.

Let's look at it in reverse. If you stop drinking one soda per day and instead drink a bottle of water, you could *lose* 30 pounds of fat in one year. Just like that. Without doing anything else different.

Have I blown your mind yet?

Just by eliminating sugary drinks and reducing your body fat, you also reduce your risk of diabetes, inflammation, and other lifestyle diseases. Double win!

Read the label before deciding whether a drink will help or hinder your health goals.

What About Sugar-Free Sodas?

Beverage companies would like you to believe that drinking sugar-free sodas is a guilt-free way to enjoy their products. Hear me now – many of them are poison! Instead of sugar, they are sweetened with chemicals such as aspartame and sucralose. A 2023 review of twenty-one studies found that artificially sweetened beverages can affect health in multiple ways, including mental health, child neurodevelopment, heart disease, kidney disease, cancer, and dental cavities [99].

If you want a healthy alternative, try flavored mineral water. Go for a brand with only water and fruit as ingredients. If you see the words *flavors*, ditch them. Flavors are an umbrella term that the FDA allows for a soup of unknown chemicals [100].

At home I love sparkling mineral water with lime juice, orange juice, or my new favorite, hibiscus tea.

Workbook

Quiz

Answer True or False

1. Removing the non-compliant foods from my environment will help me stay on track.
2. Cleaning out my environment helps me psychologically because non-compliant foods will not tempt me.
3. Keeping things like chocolate, cheese, and salty snacks in the house is okay because I won't eat them.
4. Sugar-free sodas are okay because they have no sugar.

ANSWERS in Appendix

Journal

Today I learned

Today I feel

I am proud of myself today because

One thing I can improve upon tomorrow is

What is my biggest struggle right now?

Who can I ask to support me with this?

What is my main goal this week?

What does my idea of success look like next week?

What three daily actions can I take to reach that goal?

1. _____
   _____

2. _____
   _____

3. _____
   _____

Quick Tip

Throwing out unhealthy food will probably be the hardest thing you do. Give it away, put it in a locked safe, or throw it in the trash. Once it is gone, it has no power over you. Be proud that you took this significant step. Now go shopping and get yourself some yummy healthy food.

CHAPTER 10: What's On The Menu?

"The human body has absolutely no requirement for animal flesh. Nobody has ever been found face-down 20 yards from Burger King because they couldn't get their Whopper in time." Michael Klaper, M.D.

What's In This Chapter?

In this chapter, let's get into the details of all the yummy food you will be eating. You will learn about the delicious plant foods you can discover and why they improve your health.

Nutrient Density Versus Energy Density

Before getting stuck into what yummy foods will be on your plate, I need to borrow your brain for a minute to explain a concept: the difference between nutrient density and energy density.

A nutrient-dense food is one that, compared to its calories, has an abundance of nutrients. Let's take kale as an example. Kale is a powerhouse of B vitamins, iron, calcium, potassium, vitamin C, vitamin K, and fiber, and is almost 90% water [101]. So, you can eat a lot of kale and ingest very few calories whilst getting a load of nutrients. Kale clocks in at around 40 calories per 100gm (181 calories per pound).

An energy-dense food has many calories compared to the nutrients it provides to your body. Let's take french fries as an example. Fast food fries pack about 323 calories per 100gm (1463 calories per pound)! This book promotes nutrient-dense foods and discourages most energy-dense foods. Let's do a quick quiz.

Which of these foods is energy-dense? Banana, tomato, or candy bar? If you guessed the candy bar, you would be correct. Candy can contain many calories, sugar, and fat but not much nutrition.

Which of these foods is nutrient-dense? Spinach, a soda, or a cupcake? If you guessed spinach, you would also be correct. Those green veggies have tons of nutrients but very little energy (calories).

What does this mean for you? It means you can eat a truckload of spinach and get fantastic nutrition without many calories. You can literally eat spinach till you explode and still not put on any weight. (Okay, maybe not literally. Please don't try that.)

Are you going to eat only bucketloads of spinach? No way! Because that would be boring, and you would hate it. Instead, you will eat a variety of nutrient-dense fresh fruit and vegetables, whole grains, and legumes until you are fully satisfied. You will not have to count calories or have mini portions. Yet, you will lose weight and reduce your risk of disease.

What if you want fries? Make a healthy version. Air-fried potatoes, which are very delicious, retain all their nutrients, fiber, and none of the fat of the store-bought fries. By air frying, all you do is remove the water. So, whilst an air-fried potato might have slightly more calories than a boiled potato, if you really want fries, it's the way to go.

A few foods are both energy-dense and nutrient-dense. These include nuts, seeds, and avocado, which are healthy natural foods high in nutrients but also high in fat. If one of your main goals is weight loss, it's best to minimize these foods initially. You can always add them to your menu rotation later once you have reached your goal weight.

What Foods Are On The Program?

Now that I have made you hungry by discussing fries let's look at the other yummy foods you can eat when following a healthy whole plant foods diet. They include:

- Vegetables
- Fruit
- Whole grains
- Beans and Legumes
- Herbs and spices
- Pickles, vinegar, and sugar-free, oil-free condiments, dressings, and sauces
- Sugar-free jams and preserves
- Water, tea and coffee

I created a graph so you can see the energy density of each food group. As you can see, all the foods on the left have a low energy density, and the ones on the right have a high energy density. The foods on the left also have a high nutrient density, while most on the right have a low nutrient density (with nuts, seeds, and avocado being the exception). To make your food choices super simple, you will want to consume a lot of food from the grey columns on the left and avoid* the food from the black columns on the right. NOTE: *Avocado and store-bought hummus are healthy medium density foods. Eat them sparingly if weight loss is your goal.

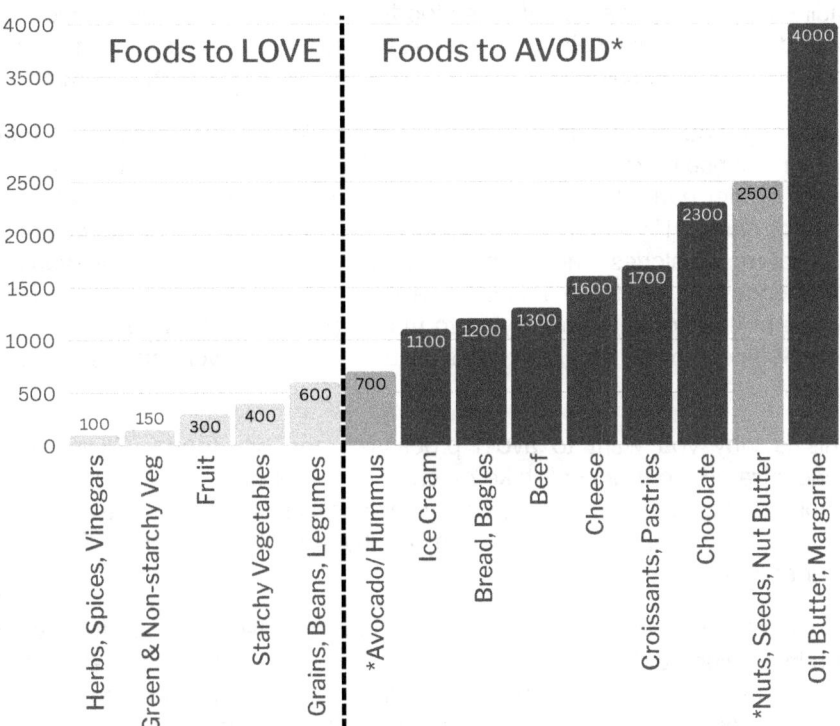

*Notice the nuts, seeds and nutbutters are on the far right. This doesn't mean that they are inherently unhealthy. They are healthy whole foods, but they should be eaten sparingly. I'll talk more about them soon.

Why Are The Foods On The Left The Only Ones On The Program?

An average person eats between three and five pounds (1.5-2.5 kg) of food per day depending on their height, weight, age, activity level, and a whole host of other variables. But let's, for this example, suggest that the average person eats around four pounds (about 2kg) of food per day. Let's also assume that this person needs 2000 calories daily to maintain weight.

If that person ate four pounds of kale, they would consume 720 calories daily. However, if they ate four pounds of french fries, they would consume 12,320 calories!

Dividing the daily 2000 calories by 4 pounds equals 500 calories per pound. So, if they eat food containing 500-600 calories per pound, they will maintain their weight easily. If some of those foods contain less than 500 calories per pound, they will lose weight. This holds true for most people. Stick to foods less than 500-600 calories per pound, and you will lose weight. It's math.

Each day, you will eat four pounds of food. So why not make that food nutrient-dense for maximum nutrition with fewer calories? Despite years and years of diet gurus trying to tell you otherwise, you cannot mess with the laws of nature. If you eat fewer calories than you burn, you lose weight. If you eat more calories than you burn, you put on weight. Now, before you get all sciencey on me, there are some caveats to that rule that go beyond the scope of this book (I'm not trying to make sports scientists out of you just yet). Suffice it to say, let's run on this assumption: Eat fewer calories and lose weight.

This is why you want to avoid processed and oily foods. Oil is highly concentrated, so it doesn't take much of it in your stomach to add up to a whole lot of calories. Those are empty calories with little nutrient value. When you are actively trying to maintain a healthy weight, added oil is thwarting your efforts.

Your goal is to fill your stomach with nutritious and delicious food that keeps you in a calorie deficit, allowing you to be full and satisfied while still losing weight. Who doesn't want that? It might take some experimentation to adapt your recipes, but this way of eating will soon be second nature, and you will wonder why you ever ate differently.

If you are breaking into a cold sweat right now, take a breath. There are recipes at the back of the book for you to try. You can combine foods for delicious meals that your whole family will love. Don't worry – you will not starve. Just the opposite. Even though it might seem scary initially, this way of eating is quite simple, and I know you can do it!

Veggies

At the risk of sounding like a broken record, eating vegetables has so many benefits. Veggies are packed with phytonutrients, vitamins, minerals, antioxidants, fiber, and water. Because vegetables are so hydrated, they are very low in calories. Eating more vegetables lowers your risk of death. You have a 26% reduced risk of early death if you eat five servings of fruit and veggies daily. For every daily serving of veggies, your risk of death decreases by 5% [102]. If that doesn't get your attention, how about this? Veggies also reduce your risk of cardiovascular disease, stroke, cancer, and diabetes. The World Health Organization says people should eat a combined five servings (approx 450gm/1lb) of daily fruit and vegetables. But you, my friend, will double that. You will aim to eat at least two pounds daily.

Starchy Vegetables

Starchy vegetables include potatoes, sweet potatoes, other tubers, corn, pumpkin, and, to a lesser extent, carrots and parsnips. Starchy vegetables are the key to being consistent with your new lifestyle. Potatoes are so versatile and filling. You can bake, boil, mash, scallop, air fry, or add to soups, stews and casseroles. Potatoes come in many varieties and colors, so try them all and find your favorites. You are seriously missing out if you are not eating potatoes multiple times per week.

Non-starchy vegetables

Non-starchy vegetables are all the other vegetables. Non-starchy vegetables have very low energy densities, so they are the healthiest foods to eat. They consist mostly of water, fiber, and nutrients, so you can eat them as much as you like. The most highly nutritious non-starchy vegetables are green leafy vegetables such as kale, collards, spinach, arugula, and chard. Eat these with gusto every day. If you are not a fan, ease yourself in by chopping them finely and adding them to spaghetti sauce or soups. You will obtain all their benefits without gagging on a mouthful of greens. I add kale to every smoothie I make. I can't taste it, but I know it's improving my health.

Eat The Rainbow

The color of the vegetables represents the nutrients they contain. Most red fruit and vegetables have similar nutrients as do most blue and green ones. The aim is to eat all the colors of the rainbow to ensure you get all the nutrients your body needs. Color coding of fruit and vegetables makes eating the rainbow easy. What if you don't like red peppers? No stress, eat a tomato instead. Not keen on purple beets? That's okay, have a purple sweet potato or an eggplant instead.

Whole Grains

Grains are the seeds of grass species such as oats, wheat, rice, millet, and quinoa, to name a few. Within your four pounds daily food intake, aim for about a quarter of each plate to be cooked whole grains. A whole grain has not been processed so its outer layer, or bran, remains intact. Bran has most of the grain's dietary fiber, vitamins, and minerals. That is why eating whole grains and avoiding refined grains is important.

Refined grains have had the bran removed, leaving just the insides, called the endosperm. Refined grains include white rice and white flour which are made into pasta, cakes, cookies, crackers, and hot dog buns. They have minimal fiber or nutrients and have no place in a healthy diet.

Whole grains, on the other hand, are very healthy. They are packed with B vitamins, vitamins A, E, and K, protein, healthy carbohydrates, and fiber. Some of the fiber in whole grains gets fermented in the lower intestine (colon) and forms short-chain fatty acids. These, in turn, reduce the risk of colon cancer [103]. Whole grains can improve your cholesterol [104] and lower your risk of type 2 diabetes. For every 50gm per day of whole grains eaten, your risk of developing type 2 diabetes decreases by 23% [105].

It's simple to incorporate whole grains into your lifestyle. Swap white rice and white pasta for brown rice and whole-grain pasta. Avoid processed cakes, cookies, and crackers; instead, make healthier versions at home. Experiment with different grains instead of rice. Try farro, barley, quinoa, or millet. Whole grain oats with berries for breakfast are delicious.

Flour

Before white flour was processed, it was lovely whole grains. To make white flour, the fiber and most nutrition are removed. Then, the grains are ground, so they become very easily digestible. Sometimes, they are even bleached. White flour, also called all-purpose flour, unbleached flour, or plain flour, is used to make cakes, pies, and pastries—which usually also contain fat to hold the flour together. Additionally, these foods generally contain added sugar to make them taste yummy. So, it's a hard NO to white flour.

Stone-ground sprouted organic whole grain flour is an ingredient I use on occasion to make pancakes and banana muffins. The recipes at the back of the book can be incorporated into your lifestyle without jeopardizing your health goals. But remember that ground flour is much more energy-dense than the whole grain equivalent, so use flour sparingly and rarely.

A Note About Bread

Bread has between 1100-1200 calories per pound (2400—2600 calories per kg). It is made from processing grains, and then other ingredients are added. Even the best organic sourdough still has 1100 calories per pound. Think also about what goes on top of the bread: butter, chocolate spread, deli meats, cheese—all the things detrimental to our health.

Have you ever tried sweet potato toast? A slice of baked sweet potato in the toaster has half as many calories as a slice of bread. Top it with mashed banana and cinnamon, and it's almost like dessert! Yum. Which are you going to choose?

If you make bread at home, use organic stone-ground sprouted whole grains, sourdough culture, and water. That is a recipe for good bread, and it's delicious. However, most bread in stores is full of additives, sugar, bleached flour, pesticides, chemicals, whey (yes, they put milk products in bread), and all sorts of nasties. It is high in calories and low in nutrition.

If you can make or purchase bread without those ingredients, a little bread will not hurt you. When I buy bread, I buy Food For Life Ezekiel® muffins which are made from sprouted whole grains. Bear in mind, all bread is calorie-dense and can slow down weight loss.

Fruit

Just like vegetables, fruits are powerhouses of flavor and nutrition. And just like vegetables, they are filled with vitamins, minerals, phytonutrients, fiber, and water. They also have some sugar in the form of fructose. Fructose does not raise your blood sugar like glucose, as the liver processes it and restores your glycogen stores for later energy [106]. If you have ever heard on the internet that fructose is bad for you, those claims are not referring to fructose in fruit. The 'bad' fructose is a component of corn, highly processed into high fructose corn syrup, or HFCS. HFCS is a sweetener used in sugary drinks and ultra-processed foods. Consumption of HFCS has been implicated in the progression of many diseases, including type two diabetes, high blood pressure, and heart disease [107]. Fructose from fruit is not the same as high fructose corn syrup. A small percentage of people on earth have hereditary fructose intolerance. For those people, eating any fructose can be fatal. For everyone else, fruit and natural sugar fructose is not a problem and should not be avoided.

Fresh or Frozen?

Do you think that fresh fruit is better than frozen fruit? Maybe yes, maybe no. If you have a blueberry bush in your garden and you eat your blueberries at the time of picking, then you can't get much fresher than that. But if you buy your blueberries from the supermarket, they are sometimes grown thousands of miles away, packaged, shipped, and then sat on the supermarket shelf. They could be two weeks old or more before you get them.

On the other hand, frozen blueberries are picked, frozen, and packed usually on the same day. So, whilst they may not have the crunch of a fresh blueberry, frozen berries generally retain more nutrients than the transported fresh ones. Frozen berries and other fruit are available all year round when you might not be able to buy their fresh varieties. Don't be afraid of frozen fruit. It is usually cheaper than fresh and is very convenient.

Cans/Jars

If frozen fruit is good, what about canned fruit? Or fruit in jars? There are a few things to look out for when purchasing preserved fruit. The first is the type of container. Glass is a great food container as it does not contaminate the food inside. Steel cans, however, can contain a chemical called BPA (bisphenol-A), which can leach into the food and cause problems in our bodies. BPA contamination can disrupt our hormones and has been implicated in birth defects, inflammation, and central nervous system dysfunction [108]. When buying cans of fruit (or any food), please look for the BPA-free certification.

The next thing to look for is added ingredients. Preserved fruit should only contain the fruit and some fruit juice. When the ingredients list any kind of syrup, put that can back on the shelf. I will discuss how you can become a food label-reading ninja in Chapter 12.

Beans and Legumes

Beans beans are good for your heart. The more you eat, the more you fart!

Some people shy away from beans and legumes because they are concerned about added gas. When you eat beans, their soluble fiber remains undigested until it reaches the large intestine. This fiber is a favorite food for gut bacteria in the colon. Gas is released as they eat the fiber and convert it to short-chain fatty acids, sometimes at embarrassing moments. Don't be afraid of beans. They are full of nutrients, including protein, iron, folate, potassium, magnesium, and healthy fiber. They are very low in fat and, like all plants, cholesterol-free. There are over 20,000 different types of legumes, so if you don't like one bean, you can spend your life trying different ones. Like whole grains, aim for about a quarter of each plate to be cooked beans or legumes.

If you cannot stomach beans and legumes right now, add just a few to your meals. Rather than making a large bean burrito, try a salad with a few chickpeas sprinkled on top. Rather than sitting down to a steaming hot bean chili, add a few black beans to a soup. Start slow and low. Fermented beans such as tempeh or natto may be gentler on your stomach than canned beans. Keep a food diary of which beans your body can tolerate and which give you the worst gas. Only you can know which beans will fall in love with your gut.

Herbs, Spices and Condiments

Knowing how to season your food with herbs and spices will elevate your meals. Like any new skill, learning about combinations of herbs and spices can take time, but the payoff is enormous. You may feel your meals are a little bland as you forgo salt. This is where herbs and spices come in. You don't even need to know about flavor combinations. For example, I'll use a salt-free pre-made Mexican blend for all my Latino food. It's got chili, oregano, lime, cilantro, peppers, cumin—all the flavors that make Mexican food so delicious. It makes seasoning so easy. Likewise, I have an Italian blend, a Cajun blend, and a Mediterranean blend. These are a great starting point. As you become more confident in the kitchen, you can learn how to use individual herbs and spices to make up your own favorite blends.

> **A note about chili:**
> If a recipe calls for chili, but you cannot handle the heat, just leave it out. Or test the waters with a quarter of the recipe's measurement and see how you go. Chili adds a flavor complexity to food you can't beat. It's worth experimenting with spice, as it opens up a whole new world of deliciousness.

Condiments can also be used with abandon, as long as they are ASOUPAS compliant. For example, a popular tomato ketchup brand contains 75% added sugar, so it is off the menu. Find tomato ketchup with no added sugar or salt instead. It takes a little bit of sleuthing in your supermarket (or online) to find the brands that meet your new high standards of culinary excellence. After you have chosen your favorite brands, just keep buying them. Some brands of condiments I like are Well Your World (wellyourworld.com/?aff=29) and California Balsamic (californiabalsamic.com/fabuloushealth). Primal Kitchen is a supermarket brand I also like. Not all Primal Kitchen products are plant-based, and some contain oil, so always read the label.

Condiments I use regularly include balsamic vinegar, olives, pickled onions, mustard, pickles of all types (make sure they are sugar-free), ketchup, and BBQ sauce. Mayonnaise and creamy dressings are often based on oil. Some salads or sandwiches need a little mayo, so I have included a tofu-based mayonnaise recipe at the end of this book. You may want to use other condiments, sauces, and dressings but cannot find a healthy version in stores. In that case, search a recipe and adapt it until you are satisfied with the taste. Home-made is generally best anyway.

Nuts and Seeds

I love nuts and seeds. They are healthy whole foods. They have the highest energy density of any whole food, so eat them in moderation. 30gm (1ounce) of walnuts daily is recommended to supply your body with healthy omega-3 fats. Walnuts can lower inflammation and are great for your brain and your heart. Adding pepitas or slivered almonds to your salad for some extra crunch may help you stay with this way of eating, but do so sparingly. Don't eat the entire bag.

What About Coffee?

Coffee is the only stimulant accepted by the Olympic Committee and other professional sports organizations during competitions. It's calorie-free and gives you a great boost before a workout. That said, coffee shop concoctions are off the menu unless you get an espresso or an Americano (black coffee).

You can top your coffee with unsweetened plant milk, but all sweeteners, flavorings, and whipped toppings are out. They are full of sugar, and trust me, you do not want them in your life. Say goodbye to the double choc caramel Frappuccino with whipped cream. It's just another culprit to add to your un-friend list. There is nothing wrong with starting your day with a soy or almond latte, so if you love a morning coffee, continue to enjoy your cup of joe.

Healthy Foods List (not exhaustive)

The world of whole plant foods is full of delicious options to try. I've made a shortlist on the next few pages. Feel free to add any of your favorites I may have missed. If the list seems daunting, don't stress. Highlight the foods you already eat and enjoy, and use them as a starting point to make meals you are familiar with. Then, experiment with new foods to add variety. Take it one step at a time.

FRUITS	VEGETABLES	WHOLE GRAINS	LEGUMES	CONDIMENTS
Apples	Artichoke	Amaranth	Adzuki Beans	Allspice
Apricots	Arugula (Rocket)	Barley	Alfalfa	Apple Cider Vinegar
Bananas	Asparagus	Brown Rice	Anasazi Beans	Bay Leaves
Blackberries	Bamboo Shoots	Buckwheat	Appaloosa Beans	Balsamic Vinegar
Blueberries	Beets	Bulghur	Asparagus Beans	BBQ Sauce
Cantaloupe	Bell Peppers (Capsicum)	Einkorn	Awasi Miso	Cajun Seasoning
Cherries	Bok Choy	Farro	Azufrado Beans	Cardamom
Dates	Broccoli	Fonio (Millet)	Bayo Beans	Chili
Dragonfruit	Brussel Sprouts	Freekeh	Black Beans	Chipotle Pepper
Durian	Butternut Squash	Kamut	Black Chickpeas	Cinnamon
Feijoa	Cabbage	Kañiwa	Black Eyed Peas	Coriander (Cilantro)

FRUITS	VEGETABLES	WHOLE GRAINS	LEGUMES	CONDIMENTS
Figs	Carrot	Millet	Black Lentils	Cumin
Gooseberries	Cauliflower	Oats	Black Soy Beans	Curry
Grapes	Celeriac	Popping Corn	Bolita Beans	Dill Pickles
Guava	Celery	Quinoa	Borlotti Beans	Dried Mushrooms
Honeydew	Collard Greens	Red rice	Brown Lentils	Fajita Seasoning
Jackfruit	Corn	Rye	Broad Beans	Garam Masala
Kiwi	Cucumber	Sorghum	Butter Beans	Garlic
Kumquat	Daikon Radish	Spelt	Canary Beans	Ginger
Lemon	Eggplant	Teff	Cannellini Beans	Gochujang Paste
Lychee	Fennel	Triticale	Chickpeas (Garbanzos)	Harissa
Mandarin	Green Beans	Wheat	Cowpeas	Hoisin Sauce
Mango	Hearts of Palm	Wild Rice	Edamame	Hot Sauce
Nectarine	Horseradish		English Peas	Italian Herbs
Olive	Jalapeño		Fava Beans	Ketchup
Orange	Jicama		Green Lentils	Lemon/Lime Juice
Papaya	Kabocha Squash		Great Northern Beans	Liquid Smoke
Passionfruit	Kale		Hyacyinth Beans	Maple Syrup

FRUITS	VEGETABLES	LEGUMES	CONDIMENTS
Peach	Kohlrabi	Kidney Beans	Mustard
Pear	Kombu	Lima Beans	Nut Butters
Pineapple	Leek	Mung Beans	Nutmeg
Plum	Lettuce	Natto	Nutritional Yeast
Quince	Mushrooms	Navy Beans	Oregano
Raspberries	Mustard Greens	Orca Beans	Peanut Powder
Rhubarb	Nori (Seaweed)	Otebo Beans	Pepper
Satsuma	Okra	Peanuts	Pesto
Strawberries	Onion	Pigeon Peas	Pico de Gallo
Watermelon	Pak Choi	Pink Beans	Pickled Ginger
	Parsnip	Pink Lentils	Red Wine Vinegar
	Peas	Pinto Beans	Rice Wine Vinegar
	Potatoes	Potato Beans	Soy Sauce
	Pumpkin	Puy Lentils	Sriracha
	Radicchio	Rattlesnake Beans	Tahini
	Radish	Red Beans	Tamari
	Romaine Lettuce	Red Lentils	Teriyaki Sauce

VEGETABLES	LEGUMES	CONDIMENTS
Runner Beans	Roman Beans	Truffles
Rutabaga	Salugia Beans	Wasabi
Runner Beans	Roman Beans	Truffles
Rutabaga	Salugia Beans	Wasabi
Scallions	Snow Peas	Wholegrain Mustard
Shallots	Soy Beans	
Silverbeet	Tempeh	
Sorrel	Tofu	
Spaghetti Squash	Trout Beans	
Spinach	Turtle Beans	
Sugar Snap Peas	Vallarta Beans	
Sweet Potato	Vaquero Beans	
Swede	Winged Beans	
Swiss Chard	Yellow Lentils	
Taro	Yin Yang Beans	
Tomato	Yuba	
Turnip		
Watercress		
Yam		
Zucchini		

There are probably foods you have never been exposed to on this list. Open your computer browser and search for *plant-based recipe for (new food)*. You will find a lot of exciting and delicious recipes to try. If you are feeling brave, delve into the murky pool of AI and ask Chat GPT™ to create a recipe using specific ingredients. Hey—you only live once!

You might not like every food on the list above, but try everything once; you may find some new favorites.

Food Swaps

Just because you are changing your health does not mean you need to miss out on flavor and your favorite foods. You just need to swap them for healthier versions. For example, did you know that just fourteen corn chips have 140 calories but only weigh 30g?

140 calories of apples weigh about 300g

140 calories of carrots weigh about 340g

140 calories of broccoli weighs about 410g

Do you see my point? Why eat 30g of corn chips when you could eat almost half a kilo of broccoli? What would fill you up more?

That may not be the best comparison. Sometimes, you want something crunchy and corn-chippy. I know when you are hankering for a corn chip, a broccoli floret will not cut it. Hear me out. How about you make your own corn chips? Instead of a bag of oily snacks, cut up some corn tortillas and bake them in the oven or the air fryer. (Be careful; they only take four minutes in the air fryer.)

140 calories of store-bought corn chips = 30g

140 calories of home-made baked corn chips = 72g

So, you can eat almost three times as many corn chips for the same amount of calories. YES PLEASE! So where are those extra calories coming from? Half the calories in the pre-packaged corn chips are not corn chips at all – they are from the oil they are cooked in. YUK!

Let's look at some other swaps.

Non-Compliant Food	New Food	Make Your Own
Jam with sugar	100% fruit preserve	Mix berries with chia seeds and some date powder
Peanut butter	PB2 defatted peanut flour	Blended peanuts
Cream/whipped topping	Pear cream	Blend canned pears with rolled oats till creamy
Fries	Air-fried fries	Air fry sliced potatoes at 400 degrees for 20 minutes
Cheese	Plant-based cheese sauce	See the recipe in Chapter 26
Mashed potatoes with butter	Garlic mash	Cook potatoes in vegetable stock; add garlic, nutritional yeast, and spices. Mash till smooth.
Soda and Fizzy Drinks	Club soda and lime juice, orange juice, lemon Juice	
Oil for sautéing	Water, vegetable stock	
Sugar	Bananas, sweet potato, dates, apple sauce	
Store-bought corn chips	Corn tortillas	Baked at 400°F for 3-5 minutes.
Potato Chips	Air-fried potatoes	Slice potatoes with a mandolin. Pat dry. Season to taste and air fry or bake at 400°F for 4 minutes.

Plant Protein

There is one question that every plant-based eater hears incessantly, and that is, "Where do you get your protein?" Perhaps you are pondering this question yourself. Well, the answer is "Everywhere!". But before I explain that answer, allow me a minute for a small biochemistry lesson.

Proteins have thousands of actions in our bodies, from creating muscle tissue to digesting food and making hormones. Proteins are indispensable, so it's no wonder that people are fixated on getting enough. All proteins, regardless of their function, comprise amino acids. Think of a protein as a building and the amino acids as the bricks that make up the building. Just like you can erect many different types of buildings using different bricks, the body can also make different proteins from combinations of various amino acids.

There are twenty different amino acids. Eleven can be synthesized in our bodies, but nine cannot. You need to get these nine 'essential' amino acids from your food [109]. In the olden days (twenty years ago), people used to think that meat was the only 'complete protein' and that plant foods were somewhat deficient in various amino acids. Nutritionists even suggested combining different plants (such as rice and beans with distinct amino acid profiles) to create a complete protein. Now we know that this is not necessary. Hear me loud and clear. All plant foods contain all the nine essential amino acids. I'm going to repeat it, but louder.

ALL PLANT FOODS CONTAIN ALL THE NINE ESSENTIAL AMINO ACIDS! (Sorry for shouting).

Some plant foods contain smaller amounts of amino acids than others, but this is not a problem as the body does not keep a score with every bite. For example, an apple's most abundant amino acid is leucine, but apples have very little cystine. (Notice how all the amino acids end in 'ine.') Oatmeal, however, has lots of cystine. So, when you have oatmeal with apple sauce (mmm) for breakfast, you get enough cystine. You do not need to count your amino acids or combine certain foods; you just need to eat a wide variety of plants. All the amino acids you need for optimal health will be supplied naturally without you even trying.

Should you count protein? I don't suggest you count macros regularly. I do approve of taking a snapshot of your usual food intake and running it through some nutrient software to see if there are any discrepancies. If you discover that your current diet is low in protein, then make sure to add protein-rich foods to every meal. This is vital to maintain muscle mass and bone density, particularly if you are elderly, post-menopausal, an athlete, or trying to put on extra muscle tissue. Here's a quick high-protein meal plan.

Breakfast:

Oats with walnuts, berries, and soy milk (high protein sources here are oats, walnuts, and soy milk).

Lunch:

Mixed veggie salad with chickpeas, tofu, and quinoa (the three high-protein sources here are chickpeas, tofu, and quinoa).

Dinner:

Stir fry with veggies, tempeh, and brown rice (high protein sources here are tempeh and brown rice).

Dessert/Snack:

Tofu chocolate mousse (tofu is a high-protein source here). This recipe is in Chapter 26.

I wrote that meal plan out in two minutes. Pretty soon, you can do precisely that—in your head—as you prepare your meals. These foods are everyday foods you may already have in your pantry and fridge. Every meal contains protein, complex carbohydrates, fiber, phytonutrients, vitamins, and minerals. Every meal is also low in fat and cholesterol-free. What's not to love?

Please don't be worried about protein. But, if you are still dubious, here's a list of the highest protein plant foods:

- Legumes—edamame, soy milk, tofu, tempeh, lentils, split peas, chickpeas, all beans
- Grains—quinoa, oats, buckwheat, spelt, cornmeal
- Vegetables—spinach, broccoli, Brussels sprouts, mushrooms
- Fruit—guava, avocado, kiwi, blackberries, bananas
- Nuts—hemp seeds, almonds, peanuts, pumpkin seeds, almonds, flax seeds

Note: Although nuts contain 15-25% protein, they can also contain up to 70% fat. So, use nuts and nut butter sparingly.

What About Protein Powder?

Many protein powders contain isolates, fillers, gums, whey, added sugars, and other stuff you don't want in your body. Buying a whole plant protein powder and using it strategically and sparingly can help you reach your protein goals. This is especially relevant for post-menopausal athletes. (Yes, if you exercise regularly, you are an athlete). Adding a scoop to your morning oatmeal or post-workout smoothie can up your protein game.

Whatever brand you decide to buy, read the ingredients label before purchasing, and buy the most whole food one you can find.

Plant Calcium

Calcium is essential for strong bones and a healthy heart. You might be mistaken for thinking that your body needs calcium from cows' milk and dairy products. You do not. Despite common perceptions, dairy products do not protect your bones against fractures. A 2015 meta-analysis of over forty studies found no association between dairy intake and fracture risk [110].

So, where do you get your calcium? Plant sources of calcium include leafy green vegetables (kale has five times more bioavailable calcium than skim milk! [86]), soy (tofu, soy milk, tempeh), millet, almonds, figs, flaxseed, sesame seeds, beans, and oats. Even mustard contains calcium. As you can see, there is no need to poison your body with bovine growth hormones in dairy products to obtain calcium.

If you want to know your calcium intake, use a food intake app that measures vitamin and mineral intake for a couple of weeks to see if you need to increase your calcium-rich foods. I recently did this and switched out my regular soy milk for calcium-enriched soy milk.

Plant-based B Vitamins

The B vitamins are a group of eight vitamins essential for cellular function and metabolism. They are water-soluble, meaning your body does not store them, so ideally, you need to get them from your food daily. There is one exception, vitamin B12, which I discussed the importance of in Chapter 6. B vitamins have both names and numbers. Briefly, they are:

B1—Thiamin. Vitamin B1 acts as a coenzyme for metabolism. This means it is a helper to make stuff happen. B1 is essential for the growth and function of cells. B1 is found in whole grains, soy milk, legumes, and nuts.

B2—Riboflavin. Vitamin B2 is also a coenzyme necessary for cell growth and energy production. It also helps break down fats and medications. B2 is found in whole grains and brewer's yeast (Vegemite and Marmite).

B3—Niacin. Vitamin B3 is central to the metabolism of glucose, alcohol, and fat. It can act as an antioxidant and help repair DNA. B3 is found in peanut butter, mushrooms, and cornflakes. Your body can make niacin from the amino acid tryptophan.

B5—Pantothenic Acid. Vitamin B5 helps make Coenzyme A, which can build and break down fats. It also assists in the synthesis of neurotransmitters, steroid hormones, and hemoglobin. B5 is abundant in whole grains, legumes, peanuts, broccoli, mushrooms, sweet potatoes, tomatoes, and kale. If you eat plants, you are probably eating vitamin B5.

B6—Pyridoxine. Vitamin B6 assists enzymes that metabolize amino acids, the building blocks of protein. It also helps make the happy hormone, serotonin, and other neurotransmitters. B6 is found in bananas, spinach, dark leafy greens, avocados, and potatoes. Some B6 can be stored in muscles.

B7—Biotin. Vitamin B7 helps break down the macronutrients, fat, protein and carbohydrates. B7 is found in avocados, sweetcorn, watermelon, whole grains, sweet potato, and nuts and seeds. Our gut bacteria also produce some biotin.

B9—Folate. Vitamin B9 breaks down a chemical called homocysteine, an amino acid that can harm the body in large amounts. B9 is essential for growth and development, especially for fetuses. It helps synthesize DNA and is used in blood cell production. Some staple foods, including bread and breakfast cereals, are fortified with folate to help prevent birth defects caused by folate deficiency. You can get B9 from green leafy vegetables, whole grains, seeds, beans, and fortified foods.

B12—Cobalamin. B12 is crucial to human existence. It maintains the myelin sheath on nerves, which protects the nerve and helps transmit information to the brain. Without B12, this sheath can break down, leading to permanent and irreversible neurological problems. B12 is also vital for DNA synthesis and the metabolism of short-chain fatty acids, which is essential for gut health. I cannot stress enough how important vitamin B12 is.

Vitamin B12 is produced by bacteria found in soil, as well as in the guts of animals. Traditionally, humans and animals would obtain B12 from consuming plants grown in soil or eating animals who grazed on plants. However, due to modern agricultural practices, soil quality has deteriorated in many places, decreasing the natural bacterial content that produces B12. This has made soil a less reliable source of vitamin B12. Many people think they need to eat meat because meat contains vitamin B12. However, because there is no longer a reliable source of vitamin B12 on earth, livestock also need vitamin B12 supplementation. The only reason meat has B12 is because the cows are given B12 supplements! Given the dangers of animal products to human health, it is much healthier to take a vitamin B12 supplement than to eat a cow.

Some plant-based food contains vitamin B12 only because it has been fortified. Look for plant-based milk, nutritional yeast, meat substitutes, mushrooms, and tempeh with added B12. Be aware that these foods are not reliable sources of vitamin B12. B12 has a low and variable absorption rate, so food sources alone may not meet your needs. Please take a vitamin B12 supplement daily. This is non-negotiable for your health and well-being!

Gluten-Free

The controversy about gluten continues. Some people avoid gluten, and they feel better. But why are they avoiding gluten? A small percentage of people, about 1%, are gluten intolerant. These people have celiac disease. A peptide in the gluten can damage their intestines, making absorption of nutrients difficult. People with celiac disease cannot ever eat gluten, or they become very ill. But what about the rest of us? Do you need gluten? You may have tried eating gluten-free, and you feel better. Did you ever stop to wonder why? Maybe it's not the gluten. Gluten is a prebiotic. It feeds the healthy bacteria in our gut. So, think carefully before you ditch it.

Think about all the places you find gluten: bread, cakes, pizza, cookies, pop tarts. Many ultra-processed foods contain gluten. So, is it the gluten that is causing your stomach upset or the other ingredients in ultra-processed food? Have you ever investigated this?

If you feel sluggish, crampy, gassy, or generally yucky after having a white bread sandwich, next time, take a look at the ingredients. Does the bread contain gums or modified starches such as maltodextrin? Is the bread organic, or has the wheat been sprayed with pesticides and herbicides like glyphosate? You will never know, as crop chemicals are never listed on food labels. Try an experiment. Next time, buy a wholegrain sourdough loaf where the ingredients are organic whole wheat or rye, culture, and salt. No additives, no chemicals. See how you feel after eating that sandwich. Remember to fill your sandwich only with whole plant foods, as the chemicals in deli meats, cheese, and other animal-based ingredients may also cause your stomach upset.

If your symptoms lessen, maybe it's not the gluten. Many people find that their gluten sensitivity goes away once they start cleaning up their diet, adding copious fresh vegetables and fruit, and leaving ultra-processed foods and animal products off their plates.

Workbook

Quiz

Answer True or False

1. The way to sustainable health is through eating many foods high in nutrients but low in energy.
2. A candy bar is energy-dense because it has lots of calories but little nutrition.
3. A candy bar is nutrient-dense because it has lots of energy.
4. Nutrient-dense foods fill you up without adding extra calories.
5. Vegetables, fruit, whole grains, legumes, herbs and spices, and nuts and seeds are the best foods for sustainable health.
6. Nuts and seeds can be used as a primary source of protein.

ANSWERS in Appendix

Journal

Today I learned
_____

Today I feel
_____

I am proud of myself today because
_____

One thing I can improve upon tomorrow is
_____

What is my biggest struggle right now?
_____

Who can I ask to support me with this?
_____

What does my idea of success look like next week?
_____
_____

What is my main goal this week?
_____

What three daily actions can I take to reach that goal?

1. _____

2. _____

3. _____

Quick Tip

Most whole plant foods are naturally low in calories and high in nutrients. If you do not want to get bogged down with science or confused by all the chatter on the internet, just stick with whole plant foods. These include vegetables, fruit, legumes (beans and lentils), and whole grains in their natural form. Nuts, seeds, and avocados can be eaten sparingly as they have high energy and nutrient densities.

CHAPTER 11: Let's Go Shopping

"There's no question that largely vegetarian diets are as healthy as you can get. The evidence is so strong and overwhelming and produced over such a long period of time that it's no longer debatable."
Marion Nestle, Nutritionist.

What's In This Chapter?

In this chapter, you will learn a simple yet effective approach to shopping so that you can keep your purchases on track and avoid falling into the trap of buying unhealthy foods.

First, let me tell you a story:

Once, there was a woman who had good intentions of eating healthier. So, she went to the supermarket to fill her cart with nutritious food. At the front of the supermarket, a lady was giving out free samples of hot dogs. Our girl was hungry, so she gobbled down a few bites. Two steps later she noticed the potato chips were 'buy one get one' (BOGO) free. So, into the cart went two family-size bags of potato chips. She made her way to the frozen section, and the store finally had her favorite double chocolate fudge popsicles in stock; Oh, heaven! She placed two of those in the cart because they are often out of stock. When she arrived at the produce section, she was overwhelmed by the variety of fresh fruit and vegetables. She didn't know what to get, so she chose a bunch of bananas and a basket of cherry tomatoes. At home, she realized she had nothing for dinner, so she ordered a pizza and scoffed a pack of chips as she waited for the delivery driver.

Does this scene sound familiar?

The supermarket can be a minefield, with all those shiny packets of cookies, pre-made easy dinners, and delicious bakery aromas wafting throughout the air. But fear not, I can help you navigate the supermarket like a pro.

The first step before you set foot in the supermarket is to have a plan. Yes, I'm serious. You must have a plan unless you want to walk out with a family-size bag of gummy worms and a gallon of chocolate ice cream. Here's how it's going down.

Plan

Plan your meals at home. You can use the spreadsheet at fabuloushealthbook.net/bonuses or just write them out. You do not need to make gourmet chef-worthy recipes; just decide what you want to eat. You can schedule different meals daily or eat the same meal every day. It does not matter. Whatever works for you and your family. In Chapter 17, I will show you an easy way to plan and prep all your meals so that eating whole plant food meals is a breeze. But for now, assume you know what you will eat for the week.

Write

Decide what ingredients you need, and write a shopping list. If you are not crazy about meal planning, open your fridge, freezer, and pantry and look for the basics: fresh or frozen vegetables and fruit, greens, spices, dry or canned beans, whole grains, and condiments. Put whatever you need for the coming week on the list. If M&Ms are on the list, remove them.

Eat

Before you go to the supermarket, eat a healthy meal or snack. This is imperative. Going to the supermarket on an empty stomach is a recipe for disaster. At the first glimpse of the sample lady, you will be reaching for a toothpick before you know it. If your stomach is satisfied, whatever is on offer for free will have no power over you. Neither will the aroma of freshly baked croissants nor the chocolate peanut butter cups at the checkout. Eating first puts you in control of your stomach.

Read

Read your list. I know this sounds obvious, but I can't tell you how many times I have written a list and then forgotten to look at it in the supermarket. I'd end up with half the things on the list and a cart full of stuff I didn't need. So, read your dang list! At the store, buy only what is on the list. No more, no less. (Unless kale is BOGO!).

The Ninja Strategy

There is a method to navigating the supermarket, and it goes like this:

Bulk it – If there is a bulk section, head there first. You can save heaps of money if you buy your oatmeal, dried beans, and grains from the bulk bins. Use hygienic collection practices and check the bins for contamination before you dig in. Once, I came home with some granola full of weevils! Urgh!

Can it – Head to the canned vegetables and beans aisle. Stock up on beans, legumes, tomatoes, passata, peaches, etc. Make sure to choose single-ingredient cans with no added salt or sugar. A little citric acid is fine as it keeps the food fresh. For fruit, steer away from anything packed in syrup or with added sugar.

Condiments—Get your spices, vinegar, and oil-free dressings. Check the labels and go for ones free of added maltodextrin, guar, and xantham gum. Finding products without these added ingredients may be difficult, but keep trying. They are out there. You only need to find one brand that suits your needs. My favorite is Well Your World (wellyourworld.com/?aff=29). Their products are available only online but far superior to anything I can find in the supermarket.

Get productive—First, head straight for hard fruit and veggies such as potatoes, onions, carrots, oranges, and melons. That way, they can sit on the bottom of your shopping cart and won't squish the softer, more delicate plant foods. Then, collect the rest of your fruit and vegetables.

Lastly, pick up greens, berries, and soft fruit like bananas and peaches.

Head to the freezer – Next up are frozen berries, fruit, veggies, and pre-cooked grains. Walk past those processed ice cream sandwiches and pizzas. They are of no value to you.

The final stretch
Did you forget anything? Do you need batteries or paper towels? Get those and head to the cashier. Do not head down the potato chip aisle or look at the elaborate cake decorating section. If you like, go past the flowers and get yourself a bunch of blooms as a reward for a great shopping experience.

While waiting in the checkout queue, do something productive like check your emails. Don't look at the candy. It is evil and does not love you. Avoid eye contact with those shiny wrappers.

Success! You did it! You bought healthy food and saved money by purchasing only the items on your list and not buying highly processed junk with little nutritional value. Good for you! I'm so proud of you.

Practice this each time you shop and very soon, you will be a supermarket ninja. You will be in and out in no time with a cart full of delicious, whole plant foods.

Workbook

Quiz

Answer True of False

1. I can become a supermarket ninja by preparing a list and buying only what's on the list.
2. Following this system will save me money as I will not be tempted to buy other items.
3. Winging it and buying what takes my fancy is the best way to shop.
4. Eating a healthy meal before shopping makes me less likely to be tempted by checkout aisle candy.

ANSWERS in Appendix

Journal

Today I learned
_____

Today I feel
_____

I am proud of myself today because
_____

One thing I can improve upon tomorrow is
_____

What is my biggest struggle right now?
_____

Who can I ask to support me with this?
_____

What is my main goal this week?
_____

What does my idea of success look like next week?
_____
_____
_____

What three daily actions can I take to reach that goal?

1. _____

   _____

2. _____

   _____

3. _____

   _____

> **Quick Tip**
>
> Shopping preparation is key to purchasing power. Using a system will save money and time and keep you healthy.

CHAPTER 12: Food Labels

"If it grew on a plant, eat it; If it was made in a plant, don't." Michael Pollan

What's In This Chapter?

That quote from Michael Pollen summarises this entire book. However, sometimes packaged food can't be avoided. Sometimes, we want food in packets. So, in this chapter, let's learn how to decipher the gobbledygook that populates a food label. At the end of this chapter, you will be so good at reading labels that you can say 'yes' or 'no' to a product in seconds.

Real Food Doesn't Need a Label

My rule of thumb is to avoid processed foods that need food labels as much as possible. Fruit and vegetables don't have food labels. Why not? Let me ask you. What are the ingredients in an apple? Or a tomato? Or a bunch of kale? Fresh produce doesn't have food labels because it IS food! You don't need the FDA to tell you what an apple is.

You may want to search for healthier versions of familiar packaged foods at the beginning of your plant-based journey. When you buy packaged foods, you must become a food label reading expert. This ensures you purchase the healthiest version available. Food labels can be confusing and misleading. The front of the package may have claims such as 'gluten-free' or 'a good source of iron.' These claims do not automatically make the food healthy. So, let's look at a food label and dissect it.

Ingredients

The ingredients list is the first thing you should look at on the nutrition panel. Very quickly, you can tell from the ingredients list whether the food is for you or not.

Start with the text in bold. Allergens are usually printed in bold text. Even if you don't have any food allergies, you can quickly see if milk or eggs are in the product, as they are both allergens and will be highlighted in bold.

Then, look for animal products, oil, sugar, or salt (sodium). Animal products can be deceptively labeled. You may see words like gelatin, whey, and casein, which are all animal products in disguise. Sugar can be labeled as high fructose corn syrup, sucrose, or dextrose. Artificial sweeteners should also be avoided. Look for ingredients such as aspartame or sucralose. Oil is usually labeled as oil, palm oil, shortening, lard, or butter. I'll talk about sodium in the next section, but as a rule of thumb, if a packaged food has fewer milligrams of sodium per serving than calories per serving, it's a low-sodium food. If it has more sodium than calories, put it back on the shelf and walk away.

> *"Food labels are weird, confusing, and stupid,"* John Chrisman, Terri's husband.
>
> My hubs tries very hard to be healthy, but, like most people, he doesn't have a degree in nutrition science. So he looks at the front of the packets and sees claims like 'whole grain,' 'high in fiber,' or 'low in sugar,' and promptly puts them in his shopping cart with a smug smile. Then, when he gets home, proudly showing the products he purchased, I sometimes pop his bubble by exclaiming that they should be in the trash. As you have discovered, the gold is on the back of the packet. He was only looking at the front. Unfortunately, he fell into the trap of being duped by marketing. He accidentally bought unhealthy products, thinking they were healthy. It wasn't his fault. All the food manufacturers use this tactic to get you to buy their products.

Deciphering The Food Label

Let's look at a nutrition label and how to determine the macronutrient composition of a food. Look at the image below.

Ingredients:
Cashew Milk (Filtered water, cashews), Tapioca Starch, Locust Bean Gum, Live Active Cultures.

Live Active Cultures:
S. Thermophilus, L.Bulgaricus, L.Acidophilus, Bifidus, L.Lactis, L.Plantarum
This is not a low calorie food. See Nutritional Facts for calorie, fat and total sugar content.

Contains:
CASHEWS, COCONUT

Nutrition Facts

Serving Size: 1 Container (150g)

Calories 110   % Daily Value*

Amount per serving

Total Fat 7g	9%
Saturated Fat 1.5g	8%
Trans Fat 0g	0%
Cholesterol 0g	0%
Sodium 5mg	0%
Total Carbohydrate 5mg	3%
Dietary Fiber 1g	4%
Total sugars 1g	
Added sugars 0g	0%
Protein 3g	

*The % daily value tells you how much a nutrient in a serving of food contributes to a daily diet. 2000 calories a day is used for general nutrition advice

Serving Size: Is the serving size the entire package (as with this example), or is it half or a quarter of the package? This is important. If the serving size is half the package and you eat the whole package, all the calories (but not the percentages) are doubled.

Cholesterol: A product with more than 0gm of cholesterol contains animal products. Put it back on the shelf – this is not for you. Believe it or not, less than 1gm of cholesterol can legally be labeled as 0gm, so check the ingredients label for animal products, too.

Fat: Fat has nine calories per gram. To determine your food's actual fat content, multiply the number of grams by nine. For this example, there are seven grams of fat.

7 grams x 9 calories per gram = 63 calories

To work out the proportion of fat, divide the fat calories by the total calories and multiply by 100%. If there are 110 calories in the entire package, and 63 of them are fat, then the percentage of fat is calculated as follows:

63/110 x 100% = 57% fat

Wow! This food is 57% fat. Let that sink in. Does the label say 57% fat? No, it does not. Do not let those pesky percentages on the label fool you. Ignore them. They do not represent the percentage of fat in the food.

So, how did the manufacturer calculate the fat at 9%, and why are they allowed to misrepresent the fat content so blatantly? Are you sure you want to know the answer? It's complex.

If you read the small print at the base of the label, it says, *"The % Daily Value tells you how much a nutrient in a serving of food contributes to a daily diet. 2000 calories a day is used for general nutrition advice."* This statement generalizes that, on average, people eat 2000 calories per day. One serving of this product would equate to 9% of your fat grams for the day. This assumes that within those 2000 daily calories, you would eat about 78 grams of fat.

As you can see, this calculation is entirely arbitrary and misleading, and it does not help anyone decide at a glance whether this food is a good fit. While the label first appears to claim the food contains 9% fat, the fat content is actually 57%! You should not eat this product if you want to lose weight.

Protein: Protein has four calories per gram. Repeat the process like you did with the fat but use four calories per gram instead of nine. For this example, there are three grams of protein.

3 grams x 4 calories per gram = 12 calories of protein

To work out the proportion of protein, divide the protein calories by the total calories and multiply by 100%.

12/110 x 100% = 11% protein

Carbohydrates: Carbohydrates have four calories per gram. Repeat the process that you used with protein. For this example, there are nine grams of carbohydrates.

9 grams x 4 calories per gram = 36 calories.

To work out the percentage of carbohydrates, divide the carbohydrate calories by the total calories and multiply by 100%.

36/110 x 100% = 33% carbohydrates

Let's see if the nutrition label is correct. 57+11+33 = 101%. Giving or taking a little rounding error is good enough for me.

Sugar: Sugar is included in the carbohydrate calories. In this example, the sugar is 1 gram, which is four calories. Four out of 110 calories is about 3.6% — so not much. This product has no added sugars.

Sodium: Be careful about sodium in food. Try always to eat foods that have no added salt. Max out sodium intake at 1500mg per day. This example product has 5mg per serving, so it is a low-sodium food.

Congratulations! Now you know how to decipher a food label. Was that difficult? Tedious? Annoying? Yes, I know it is all those things. If you continue to purchase packaged food, you must understand food labels. Go to your pantry and start doing the math with the food labels on the products you already own. Get used to eliminating products quickly and easily using this method. You will soon find the products you should keep and those you can give away.

Workbook

Quiz

Nutrition Facts	
Serving Size: 1 ounce (28.35g)	
Calories 100 % Daily Value*	
Amount per serving	
Total Fat 10g	15%
Saturated Fat 5g	25%
Trans Fat 0g	0%
Cholesterol 30mg	10%
Sodium 230mg	10%
Total Carbohydrate 0g	0%
Dietary Fiber 0g	0%
Total sugars 0g	
Added sugars 0g	0%
Protein 7g	14%
*The % daily value tells you how much a nutrient in a serving of food contributes to a daily diet. 2000 calories a day is used for general nutrition advice	

Look at the nutrition label above. Then, answer these questions.

1. Is this product of plant origin or animal origin? (Hint: look at the Cholesterol)
2. What percentage of this product is fat? Choose the correct answer (10%, 15%, 90%)
3. Is this product compliant with this program?
4. If this product is not compliant, why not? Choose the correct answer (It is of animal origin and high in fat, it is of plant origin but low in protein, it doesn't have enough sodium)
5. What do you think this product is? Choose the correct answer (cheese, chocolate, nuts, bread) Hint: look at all the nutrients then eliminate the options that don't fit the nutrient profile.

ANSWERS in Appendix

Journal

Today I learned

Today I feel

I am proud of myself today because

One thing I can improve upon tomorrow is

What is my biggest struggle right now?

Who can I ask to support me with this?

What is my main goal this week?

What does my idea of success look like next week?

What three daily actions can I take to reach that goal?

1. _____

2. _____

3. _____

Quick Tip

Ignore the marketing claims on the front of food packages. Look first to the back nutrition label. If the product has cholesterol, it contains animal products. Put it back on the shelf.

CHAPTER 13: Kitchen Essentials

"One cannot think well, love well, sleep well, if one has not dined well."
Virginia Woolf

What's In This Chapter?

Do you need specialist kitchen equipment to eat a healthy whole plant foods diet? The short answer is no. The long answer is maybe. This chapter will show you the kitchen equipment that makes eating this way quick and easy.

None of these appliances are essential. If you do not have them, you can use whatever kitchen equipment you already have. When you are ready, I suggest you purchase the best appliances you can afford. You can always scour thrift stores or eBay for secondhand ones, keep an eye on department store sales, or give hints to loved ones at gift-giving times.

A well-set-up kitchen includes a set of sharp knives, a high-speed blender, a pressure cooker, an air fryer, and a microwave. A large food processor is also handy. I went years without one; now, I use it daily.

I have curated a list of my favorite kitchen appliances and gadgets on my Walmart storefront (walmart.com/global/storefront/fabuloushealth).

As a Walmart Creator, I earn money from qualifying purchases. Pop over there and see what takes your fancy. If there is a sale my store automatically updates the sale price, so you always get the best deal.

Sharp Knives

It doesn't matter what brand of knives you buy, but make sure they are sharp! If you can get into the habit of sharpening your knives at least once per month, they will always be razor-sharp and easy to use. Blunt knives cause injuries.

Vegetable Chopper

If the thought of dicing and slicing leaves you cold, invest a few dollars into a vegetable chopper. I have the Nicer Dicer Plus. It comes with different blade attachments and a storage container. You can blast through vegetable preparation quickly and you are guaranteed to have consistent sizes every time.

High-Speed Blender

There are two brands to look for in the world of high-speed blenders. Blendtec® and Vitamix™. Vitamix is the one you can buy at Costco and the one you see many influencers using online. I personally love the Blendtec. I've had my first Blendtec for over fifteen years and only had to replace the jug once. Other than that, it runs like new. I've since bought more Blendtec blenders for family members, and they love them. Check other brands if you cannot see yourself forking out up to $500 for a blender. Always buy the best you can afford.

Food Processor

I happily lived without a food processor for years. Once I bought one, I wondered how I ever lived without it. If you have a high-speed blender, a food processor is entirely optional. However, it does a few things very well that a blender cannot.

Grating and slicing — Most food processors come with blade attachments for grating and slicing. If you like coleslaw or you like to add grated vegetables to soups and stews, this can save you a lot of hand chopping time in the kitchen. For thinly sliced potatoes, the food processor does an excellent job.

Fine chopping — Blending vegetables or nuts turns them into a paste, but in the food processor, you can control how fine you want your ingredients. One of my favorite recipes comes from the the Healthy Vegan Eating YouTube channel. Their veggie ground recipe is perfect when prepared using a food processor. Not too chunky, not too mushy. If you want your textures 'just right' a food processor is the right appliance for you. Bear in mind that it will never make your hummus as smooth as a high speed blender.

Instant Pot

If you live in the USA, you have probably heard of Instant Pot. It's a pressure cooker and a multicooker. It makes cooking beans, grains, and potatoes so easy. It also acts as a rice cooker, yogurt maker, and slow cooker. I love my Instant Pot so much that I have two! If you don't have this brand in your country, look for an electric pressure cooker with multiple functions. This appliance will save you lots of time in the kitchen.

Pots And Pans

Good-quality pots, pans, and utensils are essential. Whatever you buy, please stay away from aluminum pans, as they can leach toxic levels of aluminum into your food. The same goes for Teflon.

I love cast iron for the opposite reason. Uncoated cast iron cookware gently releases iron into food safely, and can help you maintain healthy iron levels. If you suffer from low iron and do not have cast iron pans use a Lucky Iron Fish (luckyironlife.com). Simply pop this iron fish into your pan as you cook, and it will emit trace amounts of iron into your food to help raise your iron levels. Like cast iron cookware, the lucky iron fish is a safe, medication-free way to maintain healthy iron levels.

Air Fryer

The air fryer is the appliance of the twenty-first century. I love french fries, but, as you already know, I do not love oil for frying. This miraculous device allows you to have as many french fries as you want. I love the Breville® 900 series. It's an investment but well worth it. If you don't buy anything else, get this appliance. You can bake in it, roast, air fry, dehydrate, and toast. It's a marvelous machine.

A regular air fryer is a good purchase if the Breville is out of budget. Just remember that most dedicated air fryers are smaller and do not offer the functions of the Breville, however they are suitable for making fries and falafels.

Oven/Toaster Oven

If you have a Breville air fryer, you will not need an oven or toaster oven as it supports both cooking functions. Without the Breville, an oven or toaster oven is great for baking potatoes, root veggies, cookies, and falafels.

Microwave

Many years ago, people were frightened of microwaves leaching radiation into food. There is no evidence that a microwave is bad for human health. However, the electromagnetic fields used in the heating process can destroy some nutrients, such as vitamin C, in cooking. Vitamin loss occurs with any heating method, and the microwave's beauty is that it is quick, resulting in less nutrient loss than more extended cooking methods such as baking or boiling. In contrast, some nutrients are enhanced when cooked in the microwave. For example, lycopene, a tomato phytonutrient, is more bioavailable when cooked in the microwave.

The general consensus is that you shouldn't get stressed about nutrient loss from the microwave. Use it as a convenience to cook faster or to heat leftovers. The most important thing is to get fresh whole foods into your mouth, regardless of the cooking method (except for frying in oil, of course!).

Workbook

Quiz

There is no quiz for this chapter.

Journal

Today I learned
_____

Today I feel
_____

I am proud of myself today because
_____

One thing I can improve upon tomorrow is
_____

What is my biggest struggle right now?
_____

Who can I ask to support me with this?
_____

What is my main goal this week?
_____

What does my idea of success look like next week?
_____

What three daily actions can I take to reach that goal?

1. _____
_____

2. _____
_____

3. _____
_____

> **Quick Tip**
>
> You do not need every appliance under the sun. Buy a few high-quality key pieces that will serve you for years.

CHAPTER 14: Organic Vs Conventional Produce

"The single greatest predictor of a healthy gut microbiome is the diversity of plants in one's diet." Dr. Will Bulsiewicz

What's In This Chapter?

Is it better to eat only organic produce? Or is any produce better than no produce at all? In this chapter, you'll discover the pros and cons of organic versus conventionally grown plant foods and how you can maximize your health while minimizing your budget.

Why Should You Eat Organic Food?

Most people would love to eat organic food straight from their garden — the freshest you can get. I know that this is not always practical. Many of us live in apartments or don't have the knowledge or time to spend in the garden. Some of us live in remote areas and don't have access to fresh food — let alone organic fresh food. Most conventionally grown produce in America has been sprayed with pesticides and herbicides to increase yield and lower costs. However, the most significant cost of this practice is our health.

Organophosphates sprayed on food crops attack the human nervous system and have been found in large doses in children with leukemia [111]. These toxic chemicals are routinely sprayed on the fruit and vegetables offered in the supermarket.

Does that sound appetizing? Nope – not to me either.

Some crops are genetically modified to withstand this barrage of pesticides and herbicides. These crops include corn, soybeans, potatoes, squash, beets, and apples [112].

If you can afford it, please buy organic. I buy organic produce, grains, beans, nuts, herbs, and spices for these reasons. If I'm going to the trouble of fueling my body with healthy food, the last thing I want is to contaminate it with harmful chemicals. However, there is a caveat. I recognize that organic food can be cost-prohibitive, so there are ways to save money by only buying organic versions of the foods that contain the most pesticides.

The Environmental Working Group (ewg.org) releases a list of the 12 conventionally grown foods with the most pesticides called *The Dirty Dozen*, annually. They also release a list of the fifteen conventionally grown foods with the least pesticide residue, called *The Clean Fifteen*. I use this list to save money and buy the conventional versions. You can get your list here: ewg.org/foodnews/

It is available in English y Español. I buy conventionally grown bananas, citrus fruit, and anything I will peel. If I want to use citrus zest in a recipe, I buy the organic fruit.

Oats and wheat are two grains I always buy organic. Traces of the organophosphate pesticide glyphosate have been found in these grains. When you eat a whole plant foods diet, you might start eating oats, so make sure you are not also eating a lot of toxic chemicals.

You can find out more about what pesticides are found in foods by going to whatsonmyfood.org/food.jsp?food=PO

Dirty Dozen

This is the Environmental Working Group's list of the 12 fruit and vegetables with the highest levels of pesticides every year. This list may change, so check out the latest list.

The 2024 list includes:

1. Strawberries
2. Spinach
3. Kale, Collards, and Mustard greens
4. Grapes
5. Peaches
6. Pears
7. Nectarines
8. Apples
9. Bell peppers (capsicum) and hot peppers
10. Cherries
11. Blueberries
12. Green Beans

I urge you to buy the organic fruit and vegetables on this list. If you have a garden, grow your own.

Clean Fifteen

I love this list as I can purchase conventional produce without fear of pesticides. Whether my produce is conventionally grown, homegrown, or organic, I always wash it first.

1. Avocado
2. Sweet corn
3. Pineapple
4. Onions
5. Papaya
6. Sweet Peas (frozen)
7. Asparagus
8. Honeydew Melon
9. Kiwi
10. Cabbage
11. Mushrooms
12. Mango
13. Sweet Potatoes
14. Watermelon
15. Carrots

What if you cannot afford organic produce?

I agree with Dr Joel Fuhrman, author of the book *Eat To Live*, who says that the risks of not eating fresh produce because of the fear of pesticides far outweigh the toxicity risk of eating conventionally grown produce. So, eat your fruit and vegetables, organic or not. Please wash them first in a dedicated fruit and vegetable wash.

Fresh organic produce is usually more expensive than frozen organic produce. Berries, which are very susceptible to pesticide residue, are generally more economical if purchased frozen. I buy my frozen berries in bulk at a fraction of the price of fresh berries.

Workbook

Quiz

Answer True or False

1. There is no difference between organic and conventional produce.
2. Some conventional produce contains organophosphates that can be dangerous to our nervous system and have been linked to childhood cancer.
3. It's safe to buy conventional versions of the foods on the Clean 15 list.
4. When using citrus zest, use organic fruit.

ANSWERS in Appendix

Journal

Today I learned

Today I feel

I am proud of myself today because

One thing I can improve upon tomorrow is

What is my biggest struggle right now?

Who can I ask to support me with this?

What is my main goal this week?

What three daily actions can I take to reach that goal?

1. _____

2. _____

3. _____

What does my idea of success look like next week?

_____
_____
_____

> **Quick Tip**
>
> If budget or accessibility is a concern, do not worry about organic versus conventional fruit and veggies. Just buy whatever you can afford and get them into your belly.

Notes:

CHAPTER 15: Transitional Foods

"The food you eat can be either the safest and most powerful form of medicine or the slowest form of poison." Ann Wigmore—Health Advocate

What's In This Chapter?

The plant-based food sector has grown exponentially in recent years, making eating plant-based alternatives even easier than ever. Are these new foods healthy? In this chapter, we will discuss plant-based meat and dairy alternatives and how they can fit into your new way of eating.

I'm about to contradict myself. I asked you in Chapter 9 to remove all the non-compliant foods from your house. I meant it. But I also know that Rome was not built in a day, and there is some room for compromise. Some of you will ditch all the bad stuff and replace it with healthy foods right from day one. Good for you! Others may need a little time to get used to this new way of eating. That is where transitional foods come in. These foods mimic unhealthy animal-based foods you have previously eaten but are plant-based.

Transitional Foods

Transitional foods can include vegan versions of sausages, burgers, yogurt, cheese, salad dressings, cakes, and the like. But let me be very clear here. Transitional foods are just that – a short-term option to help ease you into a new way of eating. Most transitional foods are not healthy at all. They can be chock full of fat, sugar, salt, artificial colors, flavors, and other chemicals. The only difference between these foods is that they are not made from animal products. Many are highly processed and will not assist you on your health journey. Particularly if weight loss is one of your goals. It's okay to try them out, especially if you have never eaten a whole plant foods meal before. Eating these 'Frankenfoods' regularly will not help you improve your health to the extent you deserve.

Let's look at some transitional foods and compare them to their animal-based counterparts.

You can see in the table on the next page that the vegan versions of these foods are marginally healthier than the conventional versions, but they will not help you lose weight and probably won't help much to prevent or reverse disease. Use these items sparingly and not at all if you really want success.

Animal Product	Health Issues	Plant-based Option	Health Issues	Health Benefits
Beef burger	High in saturated fat, cholesterol, hormones, antibiotics	Plant-based Beef Burger	High in fat, highly processed, added salt	No cholesterol, no hormones, low in saturated fat, more fiber
Dairy Cheese	High in saturated fat, cholesterol, hormones, antibiotics, salt	Plant-based Cheese	High in fat, added salt	No cholesterol, hormones, or antibiotics
Chocolate	High in fat, sugar, hormones, antibiotics, addictive	Plant-based Chocolate	May be high in fat, sugar, addictive	No cholesterol, hormones, or antibiotics
Dairy Yogurt	High in fat, cholesterol, sugar, hormones, antibiotics, added sugar, gums, and stabilizers	Plant-based Yogurt	May be high in fat and sugar, added gums, and stabilizers	No cholesterol, hormones, or antibiotics
Chicken Nugget	High in saturated fat, deep fried, hormones, processed, high in cholesterol	Plant-based Nuggets	May be high in fat and deep fried	No cholesterol, hormones, or antibiotics, may have more fiber
Cupcake or Cinnamon Roll	High in fat, sugar, dairy, cholesterol, hormones, antibiotics, processed white flour	Plant-based Cupcake or Cinnamon Roll	High in fat, sugar, processed white flour	No cholesterol, hormones, antibiotics

The table above refers to commercially made foods readily available at the supermarket. If you learn to make some foods at home from scratch, you can avoid unhealthy ingredients and focus only on health-promoting ones. For example, I make soy yogurt from unsweetened organic soy milk with no additives. There is no healthier yogurt on the planet. It's so good. I have included instructions on how to make it at the end of this book. I've also added healthy versions of burgers, cookies, and a delicious cheese sauce. You don't need to miss out on flavor. You just need to learn a few new cooking techniques, and you can literally have your cake and eat it, too. Head to Chapter 26 for all the recipes.

Vegan Versus Whole Plant Foods Diet

There is some confusion about the difference between a vegan lifestyle and a whole plant foods diet. I was a vegetarian for almost thirty years. I gave up meat at age eighteen but didn't give up dairy and eggs. Sometimes, I was trim, and other times, not so much. Staying at my ideal body weight was always a struggle.

When I went vegan in 2015, I did not miraculously lose weight because I was still eating processed vegan foods—bread, cookies, cakes. It doesn't matter if you put dairy butter or vegan butter in a cookie—it will still have the same amount of fat, and calories.

Being vegan means that your moral compass points toward compassion. You won't buy leather shoes or handbags, nor cosmetics with lanolin or urea, or those tested on animals. You also don't use commercial fertilizers containing blood, bone, or fish meal in your garden. Whilst being vegan is noble and helps animals and the planet, it doesn't necessarily help you stay healthy. Unless you get rid of processed foods, added sugar, oil, and salt.

When I finally started eating a whole plant foods diet, I lost fifteen pounds in two months. And I kept it off. Occasionally, if I start eating peanut butter and jam on toast or succumb to the allure of some vegan cupcakes, I'll gain weight almost immediately. For me, it's very clear. A whole plant foods diet is the healthiest way to eat. No one is saying that you can never have a cupcake again. Of course, you can. You can make whole plant foods cupcakes, and they are really yummy.

Plant-based Junk Food

Unless you have been living under a rock for the past few years, you will have noticed the explosion of plant-based junk food. Everything from cookies to cakes, pizza, ice cream, and candy. Even though it might look tempting, most plant-based ultra-processed foods are no healthier than their animal-based counterparts. You can now buy plant-based chocolate bars, peanut butter cups, and ice cream. Some junk foods are already plant-based including cookies, chips, and lollies. Before you jump in the car to rush to the supermarket, remember that junk food is still junk food, whether it has animal-derived ingredients or not. These foods may be tempting to you at the beginning of your health journey, but as you become more attuned to your body's nutrition needs, you will no longer crave this rubbish. If you are finding it difficult to leave these items on the shelf, head back to Chapter 2 to revisit why you want to change your health for the better in the first place. Then head back to Chapter 9, where I give tips on removing these foods from your environment. You might not like it right now, but you will thank yourself later as you become a much healthier version of yourself.

Here are some plant-based (vegan) foods that are not your friend. After the initial transition period, try to avoid these for the sake of your health.

- Vegan chocolate and candy
- Plant-based meat substitutes
- Plant-based dairy substitutes, including ice cream, yogurt, and cheese
- Vegan cakes, cookies, breads, pastries
- Vegan quick meals and TV dinners
- Plant-based pizzas and frozen burritos
- Snack foods: corn chips and potato chips
- Anything deep fried

If I've just listed your favorite foods, know that removing them from your diet has tremendous health benefits, and the sooner you do it, the better. Very soon, you will not have the taste for them, and you won't miss them when they are out of your life. You will be so satisfied with the meals you make using whole plant foods that you won't want to eat that processed garbage anymore.

Fries

I have given fries their own section because, in America, the UK and Australia they are everywhere. In some places, like sports stadiums, sometimes they are the only plant-based option. But oil-fried fries will derail your efforts to regain your health quicker than you can say, *"Would you like fries with that?"*. YES!—we would like fries! But, no, we will not eat the oil-fried french fries. If you want crispy, crunchy fries, make them yourself in your air fryer. Air-fried potatoes, sweet potatoes, and even carrots are delicious, nutritious, and 100% whole food compliant. So eat them up, but please stay away from deep-fried potatoes.

Cupcakes

Have you seen vegan cupcakes in the supermarket? They look so yummy. Their creamy frosting begging you to buy them. STOP right there! A vegan cupcake is still a cupcake. The ones available in the store are mass-produced, highly processed, and contain ingredients to avoid. Bleached white flour, white sugar, oils, and fats—and who knows what chemicals, additives, and other yucky stuff.

Let's avoid vegan cupcakes, donuts, cookies, snack bars, and candy. Just because they're vegan does not mean they're healthy. If you want to make a cake for your birthday, search the internet for a healthy option using wholegrain flour, sweetened with fruit, and with no added fat.

Chef AJ's *Sweet Indulgence* dessert cookbook has many birthday party-worthy recipes. It's my go-to for sweet treats. There's a link in the resources section at the end of this book.

Smoothie Bowls

Have you ever gone to a food court and bought a smoothie bowl, thinking you were eating a healthy lunch? But then, 30 minutes later, you were starving, caved in, and headed to the Chinese buffet?

You can make a healthy smoothie bowl at home, but most of the ones in food courts contain added sugars and fats. Acai fruit is generally quite tasteless until mixed with a lot of sugar, and coconut yogurt contains a lot of saturated fat. Honey and maple syrup add sugar, and nuts and coconut flakes add extra fat. If acai or smoothie bowls are an option in your local food court, ask for nutritional information first. Go for it if they are made with whole food and no added sugars.

Plant-Based Meat Alternatives

Plant-based meat substitutes have come a long way. With years of research and testing, companies have created products that look and taste like meat but are made from plants. By design, they recreate the taste and texture of beef, with all its fatty, juicy mouthfeel. So, their beef-like products have quite a substantial amount of fat. New formulations have reduced the saturated fat, but these products should still be eaten only as you transition toward more whole foods, and then only rarely.

A healthier option is a bean and veggie burger made at home. My bean burger recipe is in Chapter 26.

Plant-based Cheese

Many people find one of the most challenging animal products to give up is cheese. This is because cheese contains casomorphins, which, just like their cousin morphine, attach to the pleasure receptors in our brains, making them addictive. Casomorphins are not as addictive as morphine, but they are enough to make you want to come back for more.

Most plant-based cheese is rubbish. Ingredients like coconut oil, expeller-pressed safflower oil, modified starches, and gums make up the bulk of many brands. Some brands like Miyoko's and Rebel Cheese (USA) or La Fauxmagerie (UK) use whole food ingredients such as cashews, soybeans, nutritional yeast, and cultures. These more expensive artisan cheeses are usually worth the high price tag. But again, they are primarily fat, so they should not be eaten daily. Buy a round of La Fauxmagerie brie for your Christmas table and share it with your family. Once a year is enough.

If you want to try your hand at making your own plant-based cheese, Miyoko Schinner has a fantastic YouTube channel and a couple of excellent cheese-making cookbooks including her latest release *The Vegan Creamery*.

Nooch

Nooch is the plant-based pro's way of referring to nutritional yeast. Nutritional yeast is on the pantry staples list and should be in your pantry as soon as possible. It's an inactive form of yeast, so it's no good if you want it to make bread. However, it is high in amino acids and a bunch of vitamins and minerals, including B vitamins, chromium (regulates blood glucose), and selenium (essential for normal functioning of the immune system) [113]. It adds a distinct umami flavor to recipes, which is why it gives dishes a cheesy flavor. You can purchase nooch fortified with vitamin B12, but as concentrations amongst brands vary considerably, please don't rely on it as your primary source of vitamin B12.

Head to Chapter 26 for the most amazingly delicious cheezy recipes including nooch as an ingredient: cheeze sauce, bechemal, tofu ricotta, and parmesan.

Cooking Without Oil

Oil will thwart your efforts at fabulous health. Really. If all you did was remove added oils from your diet, you would be much closer to health. Oil has nine calories per gram. That's over twice the calories as carbohydrates and protein. Unlike most whole foods, it has no water, which means it is very dense. Just one tablespoon of oil can have almost 200 calories! And it takes up a teeny tiny space in your stomach. Oil adds little nutrition to your food. It coats the tastebuds and makes it difficult for the full taste of the food to shine through.

"But the food will stick!" I hear you cry. Don't worry. I have you covered.

Most whole plant foods, especially vegetables, are water rich. As they are heated, they will release moisture. Foods like mushrooms, zucchini, and onions all have high water content. So, just throwing them into a skillet or saucepan and stirring is usually enough to stop them from sticking. If you allow them to dry fry, the pan will have a brown tinge. Before it gets burned, splash in a little water or salt-free veggie stock. This is called de-glazing. Running your spoon or spatula over the brownness will lift off the pan and form a sauce. This is where the flavor is. Keep doing this as often as necessary to keep your food from sticking. Don't throw out that sauce! Instead, drizzle it on top of your food when serving. It's delicious.

Workbook

Quiz

Answer True or False

1. I can eat as much vegan cheese and burgers as I want and still lose weight on this program because all vegan food is healthy.
2. Most transitional foods try to mimic their conventional counterparts, so they are still high in fat, salt, and sugar.
3. The main difference between animal foods and vegan versions is that the vegan foods have more cholesterol.
4. If I really want to succeed in this program, I will not make transitional foods an integral part of my diet.

ANSWERS in Appendix

Journal

Today I learned

___

Today I feel

___

I am proud of myself today because

___

One thing I can improve upon tomorrow is

___

What is my biggest struggle right now?

___

Who can I ask to support me with this?

___

What is my main goal this week?

___

What three daily actions can I take to reach that goal?

1. ___

2. ___

3. _____
_____

What does my idea of success look like next week?
_____
_____
_____

Quick Tip

Remember that plant-based meat products and other transitional foods should only be used initially. The sooner you wean yourself off processed vegan foods, the better.

CHAPTER 16: Whole Plant Foods On A Budget

"If you don't design your own life plan, chances are you'll fall into someone else's plan. And guess what they have planned for you? Not much." Jim Rohn

What's In This Chapter?

This chapter will bust the myth that plant-based eating is only for the wealthy. Whole plant foods are some of the cheapest foods available as they come straight from the farm. The less processing a food has, the less expensive it is. I'll also share simple prep hacks to help you save money and time in the kitchen.

Whole Plant Food Meals On A Budget

In Chapter 11, we went to the supermarket, and in Chapter 12, we learned all about food labels. By now, you should have a good idea about which foods to buy each week for you and your family. Let's review the most budget-friendly ways to stock your plant-based kitchen for the week.

Fruit and Vegetables

Buying in-season fruit and vegetables from your region will save you money. Look for supermarket specials and stock up on the foods with the best deals. In the heat of summer, you can buy a whole tray of mangos for the cost of a single fruit in winter. Chop them up and put them in the freezer for a supply of yummy mangos all year round. If you know how to preserve fruit and vegetables, Summer is a great time to get them cheaply.

There is no shame in purchasing frozen fruit or vegetables as long as they are not packaged with added sugar, salt, or sauces. Frozen berries, for example, are usually much cheaper than fresh ones. They won't go moldy in your fridge before you eat them and will be on hand whenever needed. Another time-saving benefit is that they come pre-chopped! My freezer is always stocked with shelled edamame, shredded potatoes, grilled corn, and mixed berries.

Beans and Legumes

Beans and legumes (lentils) are the most economical sources of protein around. Plus, they are satiating, versatile, and packed with fiber. Dried beans are about a quarter the price of canned beans. They store well in the pantry and are very easy to cook. Yes, they take a bit of preparation, but it's well worth the effort. I cook up a whole pack of dried beans in the Instant Pot, then section them into servings and store them in the freezer.

Whole Grains

As with beans, dry whole grains can be stored in the pantry in airtight containers. Like beans, some of them take a little while to cook. I'll cook up a batch of einkorn or quinoa and freeze it for later. I'm rubbish at cooking rice. I usually forget about the rice and it ends up like mush. So, I'll buy pre-cooked, frozen brown rice. It does cost more, but for me, it's better than my terrible attempts at rice cooking.

Have you tried minute rice? It's brown rice that has been precooked and then dehydrated. It seems weird, but it's awesome! Minute rice is reconstituted in just three minutes in boiling water. It is just as nutritious as regular rice but so much more convenient.

There has been some research on the potential presence of toxic compounds such as lead and arsenic in rice. Washing your rice prior to cooking and eating a variety of whole grains can reduce your exposure [114].

Herbs

Adding herbs to your cooking can really elevate the flavor of a meal. Fresh herbs are costly and tend to go slimy in the fridge after a couple of days. Growing herbs and greens is simple and economical if you have even the tiniest space in your home. You can grow an endless supply of herbs for minimal cost on your balcony or windowsill. You can use them fresh or dry them out in times of abundance for later.

Search YouTube for gardening videos (my favorites are Gardenary, Epic Gardening, and Grow Veg), and save yourself money.

Spices

If you can afford them, buy organic spices. At the very least, please purchase spices from name brands. Recently, I've read reports of 'fake' spices being sold in stores [115]. When the spice on the label is not inside the bottle, this can not only ruin your dinner but also your health. Who knows what's ground up in there? So, while legitimate spices may be costly, you can save money by purchasing refills instead of a new bottle. Many supermarkets sell spices in bags that you can use to top up your existing containers. I buy my garlic, onion, and cinnamon in pound bags and refill as needed. In case you were wondering which spices have been identified as at risk of being fake, they are oregano, black pepper, chili powder, saffron, paprika, and turmeric.

Buy In Bulk

I've only recently started buying some food items in bulk. I just don't have room for a 25-pound bag of brown rice! Plus, it would take my whole life to eat it all. But I do use the bulk bins in the supermarket. They are great for many reasons:

1. You can bring your own bags and save plastic packaging.
2. You can take as little or as much as you like.
3. You can try different foods without committing to a whole package.
4. The food is usually much cheaper than its pre-packaged counterpart on the shelves.

Bulk items to buy include wholegrain oats, nuts, grains, beans, and pasta. You can also stock up on canned tomatoes and tomato sauce whenever they go on sale.

If you have room in your home and the budget to purchase large quantities of food, please make sure that you store it in airtight containers away from any dampness and potential critters and creepy crawlies.

Pantry Staples

Some items should always be in your pantry. Even if you have nothing fresh in your fridge, you can whip up a quick meal just with pantry items. It may not be pretty, but it will be nutritious and do the job in a pinch. Never run out of these products.

A great start to your pantry includes:

- Canned tomatoes and no-added-salt tomato sauce (passata)
- Canned beans or legumes
- Tomato paste
- Roasted Red Peppers
- Vinegar (balsamic, rice wine, apple cider)
- Nutritional yeast
- Oatmeal
- Dehydrated mixed vegetables
- Dehydrated mushrooms

- Whole grain or legume pasta (any shape)
- Wholegrain or soba ramen noodles
- Herbs and spices: Get the pre-mixed ones without any additives. My favorites are Italian, Indian, and Mexican.
- Salt-free vegetable stock powder
- Miso
- Soy Sauce, Tamari, Liquid Aminos—go for the low sodium variety

For dinners that take a while to cook:

- Dried beans and legumes
- Whole grains

These items are good to have but not essential. Depending on where you live, they may be hard to find.

- Dehydrated tofu (No, it's not weird, it's a lifesaver)
- Soy curls
- Sriracha

Let's make some dinners with items solely from the pantry.

Bean Chili—tomatoes, tomato sauce, Mexican spices, kidney beans.

Minestrone Soup—dehydrated mixed vegetables, veggie stock, Italian herbs, tinned tomatoes, lentil pasta shells, and chickpeas.

Spaghetti Romesco—tomatoes, tomato paste, roasted red peppers, Italian seasoning, lentil pasta shells.

In the Freezer

The freezer doesn't have to be a graveyard for leftovers. Keep these foods on hand to make instant meals.

- Mixed vegetables
- Shelled edamame
- Pre-chopped onion
- Mixed berries
- Any frozen fruit
- Grated/cubed potatoes
- Pre-cooked brown rice or other grains

Asian noodle soup bowl. Serves 2.

This is my favorite lunch right now.

1 pack of brown rice ramen

2 cups frozen mixed vegetables

½ cup shelled edamame

1/2 block dehydrated tofu soaked in veggie stock and cubed

4 cups vegetable stock (1 tbsp stock powder with 4 cups water)

Mixed herbs of choice

Chilli (to taste).

If you don't have brown rice ramen noodles, you can use frozen, pre-cooked brown rice. Use only ½ cup of stock, and you have fried rice.

Can you start to see how easy it is to quickly make meals with these staples? You don't need fancy ingredients. Sure, if you want to expand your culinary horizons, go right ahead. There is an infinite array of plant-based influencers, all keen to get you to try their latest recipe. For me, the best way to stick to this way of eating is to forget about recipes and just throw things I like together. I have created recipes for you in Chapter 26 to get you started. Once you master these, take it to the next level by freestyling flavor combinations to create your own masterpieces.

You don't need to learn to be a chef. You just need to put together a few yummy ingredients that keep your stomach full and help you reach your health goals. The recipe police will not arrest you for having beans and veggies on top of a baked potato every night for a week. If you like it, eat it and enjoy.

Workbook

Quiz

Answer True or False

1. Eating whole plant foods is cost-prohibitive and only for the wealthy.
2. Dried beans and lentils are almost four times cheaper than canned .
3. Buying food from the supermarket bulk bins lets you try new foods.

ANSWERS in Appendix

Journal

Today I learned
_____

Today I feel
_____

I am proud of myself today because
_____

One thing I can improve upon tomorrow is
_____

What is my biggest struggle right now?
_____

Who can I ask to support me with this?
_____

What is my main goal this week?
_____

What three daily actions can I take to reach that goal?

1. _____
_____

2. _____
_____

3. _____
_____

What does my idea of success look like next week?

_____

_____

_____

> **Quick Tip**
>
> Keep your pantry and freezer stocked with the basics. Learn to make two or three easy meals and eat them on repeat.

CHAPTER 17: Be Prepared

"By failing to prepare, you are preparing to fail." Benjamin Franklin

What's In This Chapter?

In this chapter, you will learn how to set yourself up for success, including how to prepare food for the week. One of the best ways to stick to your nutrition plan is to always have food available. When the food in your fridge and cupboard is ready-to-go healthy whole plant food, you can't go wrong. Preparation beats motivation 100% of the time.

Prepping

No, I don't mean holing up in a bunker in the Nevada desert. I mean doing the bulk of the chopping and food preparation for the week ahead. Food prepping can save lots of time, but it can also backfire on you. You might make a massive pot of soup, but your family doesn't want to eat it every day for a week.

My friend Dianne Doyle from the Facebook group Plant Based Dallas introduced me to a way of prepping ingredients instead of whole meals. (Go check out the group, especially if you live in the Dallas/Fort Worth area). Dianne invites group members to fill twelve mason jars with a chopped vegetable, grain or legume. Then we all meet at her home and swap our jars. We come with twelve jars of one food and leave with twelve different foods! That's an excellent way to get prepping done in an instant. Prepping ingredients instead of whole meals saves time but also allows for meal spontaneity. Thanks Dianne!

Primary Prep—Once Per Week

If you don't have twelve friends in your area who are eating the same way as you, it's still very easy to prep your ingredients. Hubs and I usually prep all our veggies and fruit on a weekend while watching sports on TV.

First, I wash and dry my veggies, then get to chopping. I chop them into the sizes that I usually use for my meals. Onions are diced, carrots and zucchinis are sliced, and broccoli is floreted (is that a word?). Each veggie goes into its own glass canning jar and into the fridge. When I want to whip up a stir-fry, everything is ready to go, and dinner is ready in five minutes.

Then, onto the salad. There are always three or four different greens (kale, spinach, rocket, little gem, romaine), herbs (basil, cilantro, dill), radish, peppers, carrot, celery, cabbage. I call it my kitchen sink salad. Everything goes in but the kitchen sink. I leave it dry in Tupperware or a Ziplock bag. When it's lunchtime, I top with all the wet ingredients: tomatoes, cucumbers, fruit et cetera. I'll teach you my winning formula in a few pages.

Next, I cook beans, grains, and potatoes. For these, I use my Instant Pots. I have two, but if you only have one or none, you can still cook your beans, grains and potatoes on a stovetop. I love the Instant Pot because all I have to do is put the potatoes in the pot with a smidge of water, and twenty minutes later, they are done. It's a tag-team system: potatoes in one, grains in the other. Then, in twenty minutes, beans and lentils go in.

While the Instant Pots are on duty, I'm air-frying my marinated tofu and blending some salad dressings. Finally, I'll prepare a complete meal: either minestrone soup, bean chili, or spaghetti sauce. My week is prepped by the time the football is in the final quarter. I have no excuses not to eat well for the next seven days. It's so easy to create a speedy bowl of deliciousness when it's lunch or dinner time.

Secondary Prep—On The Fly

If you use up one of your jars or run out of salad, the time to re-prep is immediately or the next day. The minute you notice that you only have enough pre-cooked potatoes for tonight's dinner, get that Instant Pot cooking up a new batch. As soon as you use the grated carrots, go ahead and grate a new jar full. As the week progresses, you will eventually run out of food to fill the jars. Then it's time to go shopping again. The beauty of this method is twofold:

1. You have done most of the work on the weekend, so creating weekday meals requires less effort.
2. You can see exactly what you have prepared, so it makes choosing what to eat much simpler.

When you have brown rice, green peas, and mushrooms prepped, you can make mushroom risotto. When you have zucchini, bell pepper, and red onions prepped, you can whip up some fajitas. I love this method of prepping because it doesn't require making any recipes—it's more freestyle.

But what if you like making soups, casseroles, and lasagna? I've got a solution for you: freeze them.

Freeze It

Purchase silicone freezer trays of different sizes. They are my go-to for leftovers, but you can also use them to prep your meals into serving sizes. Make your pot of soup or casserole, then place single servings into the trays and freeze. Once frozen, pop the food out of the tray, label, and store in Ziplock bags or vacuum-sealed bags. Now your trays are empty for your next recipe. If silicon trays are unavailable where you live, try this: Let your food cool, place a labeled Ziplock bag inside a square container, fill, and freeze. When frozen, remove the container. Food that you freeze into squares stores more efficiently than food frozen in random shapes.

Snacks

Snacks are my downfall. Once, I estimated that I ate over 500 calories a day on snacks. These were 'healthy' home-made snacks, too. Imagine if I was buying unhealthy snacks from the store! Snacks can be a great addition to your healthy meals, or they can thwart all your hard work. The trick is to make your snacks as healthy as possible and eat them in moderation.

One homemade healthy oatmeal and banana cookie with your afternoon cup of tea likely will not derail your health efforts. But six? That's over 400 calories!

Some yummy snacks I eat regularly include:

- Home-made oil-free hummus and vegetables
- Fresh fruit
- Home-made tofu chocolate mousse
- Home-made oatmeal cookies
- Home-made soy yogurt
- Portioned walnuts (1oz or 30gm)

Try your best to avoid protein bars, snack bars, chips, crackers, and all the other snack foods available at the Quik-e-mart. You can always buy a banana if you are starving and away from home. Even airports sell bananas. Save yourself stress by never being without food. Bring snacks with you on trips, in your car or handbag. I've been known to carry a cooked potato in my pocket when flying. No—that's not weird.

Prepped Frozen Meals

I love pre-made dinners. If I lived alone, I'd make full meals and freeze them at the start of the week. Three minutes in the microwave, and dinner would be on the table. My Hubs detests frozen food, so that is not an option in my home. But if you prefer to make a huge lasagna or stew and freeze it for later, go ahead.

Meal Planning

If you prefer to plan your meals, a spreadsheet can be very helpful. Spreadsheets take the daily stress out of dinnertime because you decide what to eat in advance. This stops daily discussions about what to cook and prevents the temptation to order takeout after a busy day.

Create columns for the day or the week, the recipe you want to cook, and a shopping list. In the recipe column, load the URL for the recipe or, if you have a cookbook, the book title and the page number.

At the start of the week, fill in all the recipes. Then, for each recipe, check your fridge and pantry for ingredients you may be missing. Make a shopping list and buy only what is on the list. This way, you will save money and reduce food waste. If you keep one day for leftovers and another for pre-cooked frozen meals, you won't need to cook every day. Head to fabuloushealthbook.net/bonuses for a complimentary copy of my spreadsheet, with examples. Remember to copy it first, before you make any changes.

Workbook

Quiz

Answer True or False

1. Healthy plant-based eating is complex and requires many weird, hard-to-source ingredients.
2. Dehydrated or frozen vegetables are a great alternative to fresh vegetables as they are more convenient and last longer.
3. Canned beans are quick and easy. Dried beans take longer to cook, but are cheaper.

ANSWERS in Appendix

Journal

Today I learned
___

Today I feel
___

I am proud of myself today because
___

One thing I can improve upon tomorrow is
___

What is my biggest struggle right now?
___

Who can I ask to support me with this?
___

What is my main goal this week?
___

What does my idea of success look like next week?
___
___
___

What three daily actions can I take to reach that goal?

1. _____

   _____

2. _____

   _____

3. _____

   _____

> **Quick Tip**
>
> Meal planning need not be complex or rigid. Do as much or as little as suits your lifestyle. At least plan your shopping list and buy only healthy foods. You are on the right path if you have healthy food at home.

CHAPTER 18: Nutrient Loading

"I don't understand why asking people to eat a well-balanced vegetarian diet is considered drastic, while it is medically conservative to cut people open and put them on cholesterol-lowering drugs for the rest of their lives",
Dr Dean Ornish.

What's In This Chapter?

If you have struggled with maintaining your optimal weight throughout your life, the information in this chapter will be a breakthrough. Even if you currently eat a whole plant foods diet, you may still be carrying around excess belly fat that can thwart your health goals and contribute to metabolic disease. If this is you, then this chapter will change everything. Once you start using the simple concept in this chapter, the excess weight will literally fall off you. Keep reading and find out how easy it is to push through a weight loss plateau and stay at your goal weight.

Veggies For Breakfast

Yep, that's right. You will start eating veggies—for breakfast! Whaaat??? Before you run away or start crying, hear me out.

When eating veggies for breakfast was suggested to me, I thought there was no way I was going to eat veggies first thing in the morning. Oatmeal is nutritious and yummy. Why should I change? So, I did a breakfast nutrition analysis, and my oatmeal came in at over 500 calories. Eating a pound of vegetables in the morning barely hits 250 calories and really fills me up—not only with tasty goodness but also with a huge number of vitamins, minerals, and phytonutrients.

So, just by cutting out 250 calories at breakfast, you can already be in a calorie deficit for the rest of the day, whilst still getting an abundance of whole food nutrition. That's what I call winning! If you have been eating highly processed foods, sugar-laden cereals or breakfast pastries, eating veggies for breakfast might be a giant leap. Take it one day at a time. Start by eating veggies for one day per week, then two, then three, and so on. You don't need to eat veggies for breakfast every day. But you can! I eat them about five days per week, with the other two days switching between oatmeal, fruit, and yogurt.

So, how do you make those veggies tasty? Believe it or not, your taste buds will change with the increase of healthier foods exposed to them. I'm a bit lazy, so I just chop up a whole heap of my favorite veg (carrot, broccoli, zucchini, cauliflower, green peas) and put them in a container in the fridge (Go back to Chapter 17 for tips on how to ingredient prep in advance). Then, each morning, I just pop some veggies on a bed of greens (lacinato kale is my favorite) and steam them in the microwave or sauté in salt-free veggie stock on the stove. A squirt of reduced balsamic vinegar on top or a sprinkle of herbs gives you a quick, delicious breakfast.

Keep some yummy sauces on hand in the fridge or freezer. They are great for topping your veggies. Check out the recipes at the end of the book for delicious marinara sauce, mushroom gravy, or my favorite: vegan cheesy sauce. Put this book down, make some now, and be prepared for tomorrow morning's feast.

Eat Low Energy Density Foods First

Eating veggies for breakfast follows the concept of nutrient loading. The premise is that if you preload your stomach with very low-calorie food, such as salads or vegetables, your stomach has less room for more energy-dense foods. If you eat your veggies for breakfast, and then a couple of hours later you are hungry, feel free to have some oatmeal or other starchy carbohydrates. You will naturally eat fewer calories, I promise.

Sometimes, when people think of salad or veggies, they believe they will be hungry. It's true, you will not feel full if you just have a bowl of lettuce and tomatoes. Salad is not iceberg lettuce and a soggy tomato. Rethinking what salad is will change your health.

When I talk about salad, I'm describing an enormous salad chock full of greens, brightly colored vegetables, cooked grains and legumes, and delicious dressing. It's a satisfying meal that will keep you full until dinner.

From now on, for every meal you have, follow the concept of nutrient loading. Low-calorie, nutrient-dense foods first, higher calorie energy-dense foods later. How does this look in the real world?

Here is a sample day:

Breakfast

2 large handfuls of spinach, 1 pound of steamed vegetables, balsamic vinegar and spices.

Morning tea (If you are hungry)

Oatmeal with banana, blueberries, cinnamon, flax meal, unsweetened soy milk.

Lunch

A large salad with greens, carrots, beets, tomatoes, cucumber, red peppers, snap peas, boiled potatoes, and kidney beans, dressed with oil-free dressing.

Snack

Big bowl of berries and mango.

Dinner

Small side salad (leftovers from lunch), vegetable, chickpea curry, and brown rice.

Dessert

Nice cream made from frozen bananas and mango.

Did you notice how there are no measurements? No weighing? No counting calories? No counting macros? It is because you don't need to count when you eat a whole plant foods diet free from ASOUPAS. You can eat till you are satisfied with all this lovely food and still lose weight. I have included some of my go-to recipes at the end of this book so you can get started immediately.

Salad Prep Like A Boss!

I have heard the phrase "I hate salads" a hundred times. May I suggest you dislike the salads you have thus far been introduced to? May I open your mind to the world of amazing salads and ask you just to give them a try? Here's how you make the perfect salad.

1. Start with greens—all types of greens. Forget that sad iceberg lettuce. Go for rocket (arugula), baby spinach, mustard greens, kale, collards, and chard. The darker the better, and the more the better. Chop them up until they are small bite-sized pieces.

2. Add fresh herbs for bursts of flavor. My favorites are basil and cilantro, but you can add dill, oregano, or parsley.

3. Choose your favorite different colored vegetables: carrots, cherry tomatoes, cucumber, beets, celery, snap peas, red, green or orange pepper, purple and white cabbage, radish, jicama, mushrooms, broccoli, cauliflower, zucchini, onions, spring onions – whatever takes your fancy. Chop them up into bite-sized pieces too. Throw them in with the greens and herbs. Toss them about.

   The vegetables do not have to be raw. You can have a mix of roasted, steamed, and raw vegetables. There are no rules.

4. Choose your favorite fruit: apples, pears, strawberries, blueberries, oranges, mandarins, pineapple, mango. Chop them up into bite-sized pieces and toss with the veg and greens. Adding fruit to a salad is optional but I always do it. Fruit adds a sweetness that really elevates salad to the next level of deliciousness.

5. Add your favorite starches: corn, boiled potatoes, roasted potatoes, sweet potatoes, cooked rice, quinoa or farro. Throw them on top. You can even heat them first for a warm salad.

6. Add your favorite legumes: black beans, pinto beans, chickpeas, kidney beans, and brown lentils (not red, they are too squishy) – hot or cold. It's your choice.

7. Top with oil free dressing, balsamic vinegar and salt free spices.

8. For some crunch, add a sprinkle of seeds or chopped walnuts. Be careful though—these foods have very high energy densities. Add no more than 30 grams (1oz) per serving.

Notes:

1. Keep the greens and vegetables in the fridge undressed in a large airtight container.

2. Keep cooked potatoes and beans in the fridge. Then it is easy to just add your toppings of choice and customize your salad for each meal.

3. Wait until you are ready to eat the salad before adding wet ingredients, such as cucumber and chopped tomatoes, watermelon, or anything with a high water content. Storing them with your dry ingredients will make your salad soggy.

Use this salad creator with whatever you have in your fridge. Change up the veggies and dressings. The combinations are endless.

SALAD PREP LIKE A BOSS

GREENS AND HERBS
All types of greens. Go for rocket (arugula), bay spinach, mustard greens, kale, collards, chard. The darker the better. Add herbs: cilantro, parsely, basil, mint, dill.

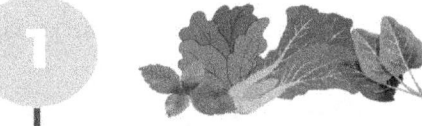

VEGETABLES
Carrots, tomatoes, cucumber, beets, celery, snap peas, peppers, radish, cabbage, jicama, mushrooms, broccoli, cauliflower, zucchini, onions, spring onions.

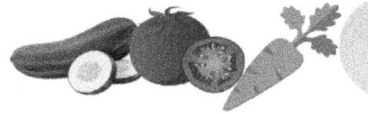

STARCHES
Corn, boiled potatoes, roasted potatoes, sweet potatoes, cooked rice, quinoa or farro. Throw them on top. You can even heat them up first for a warm salad.

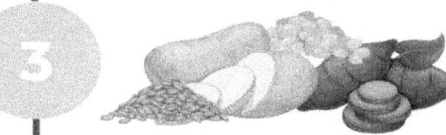

LEGUMES
Black beans, pinto beans, chick peas, kidney beans, brown lentils (not red) - hot or cold. It's your choice.

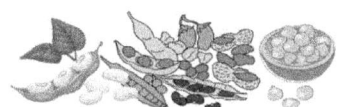

FRUIT
Apples, pears, strawberries, blueberries, oranges, mandarins, pineapple, mango. Chop them up into bite sized pieces and toss with the veg and greens.

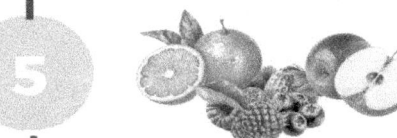

OIL FREE DRESSING
Flavored balsamic vinegar, whole food dressings,. lemon juice.

NUTS AND SEEDS
For some crunch add a sprinkle of seeds or chopped walnuts. Be careful though - these foods have very high energy densities. Add no more than 30 grams (1oz).

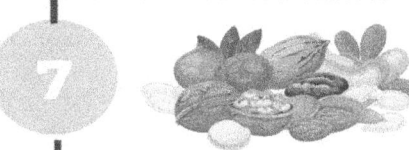

Workbook

Quiz

Answer True or False

1. Nutrient loading involves filling up on low-calorie foods before eating higher-calorie foods.
2. Eating dessert first is a form of nutrient loading.
3. You can't add fruit to a salad because fruit is only for snacks.
4. Because of the carbohydrates and sugar in fruit, I am limited to two servings per day.

ANSWERS in Appendix

Journal

Today I learned
_____

Today I feel
_____

I am proud of myself today because
_____

One thing I can improve upon tomorrow is
_____

What is my biggest struggle right now?
_____

Who can I ask to support me with this?
_____

What is my main goal this week?
_____

What does my idea of success look like next week?
_____
_____
_____

What three daily actions can I take to reach that goal?

1. _____
   _____

2. _____
   _____

3. _____
   _____

> **Quick Tip**
>
> When you fill your stomach with low energy-dense foods like greens and non-starchy vegetables, you leave less room for higher energy-dense foods in your stomach. The result? You eat fewer calories.

CHAPTER 19: How To 'Plantify' Your Favorite Recipes

"The evidence is clear: the more we consume plant-based foods, the less we are likely to suffer from heart disease, cancer, diabetes, osteoporosis, and many other chronic conditions." Dr. T. Colin Campbell

What's In This Chapter?

Transitioning to a whole plant foods lifestyle from a completely different way of eating can be daunting and overwhelming. In this chapter, I will help you take your favorite family recipes and 'plantify' them. I will teach you how to substitute ingredients to give a healthy twist to your family favorites. Will they taste the same as the old version? Maybe, maybe not. But I can promise you they won't make you sick and they won't make you fat. So leave your preconceived ideas about food at the door, and let's get cooking.

Swap It!

Do you remember back in Chapter 10, we talked about plant-based swaps? Hopefully, you have already started implementing some of these. Now, you will incorporate them into your favorite recipes. Okay, they are *my favorite* recipes, but they might be the foods you like eating too, so let's use them as an example.

When you swap out a meat ingredient, try to swap it with the healthiest alternative, usually a legume or bean, tofu or tempeh. Do not stress if, in the beginning, you are enticed by those plant-based packaged meat alternatives. Rome was not built in a day. If those meat alternatives help you stop eating meat and start eating more plants, then I'm all for it. Please use them sparingly. Eventually, you will realize that some plant-based meat substitutes are not great for your health and that whole foods taste just as yummy and are better for you. Wean yourself off them by using half meat alternatives to half beans, for example, and gradually reduce the number of plant-based meats until you no longer rely on them.

If you are ready to dive in headfirst, you can try these recipes as is or adapt them to suit your current palate.

Basic 'Plantifying' Formula

Some of your favorite meals can easily be plantified, others, not so much. Spaghetti sauce, lasagna, casseroles, and soups are easy peasy. Other recipes require more trial and error. Here's my formula to make any recipe healthier:

1. Remove the oil. Whenever a recipe says to sauté in oil or butter, sauté in either water or veggie broth.

2. Swap the meat for a plant-based option. For red meat, use brown lentils, tempeh, or beans; for white meat, use tofu. For soups, add more veggies and leave out the meat altogether.

3. Season with a lot of herbs and spices.

4. Taste, taste, taste until you are happy and satisfied.

Here are some easy ideas to get you started.

Spaghetti Bolognese

An Aussie favorite.

1. Omit the oil and sauté your onions and other veggies in salt-free veggie stock. Try the Well Your World one, which is delicious. There's a link in the resources.

2. Some people add carrots and celery to spaghetti Bolognese, but not me. If you like them, keep adding them.

3. Instead of meat mince, use either Butler's Soy Curls blitzed in the food processor to break them up, or brown lentils. (Butler's Soy Curls are available on Amazon; I have a link in the resources) For first timers, this is where you would use the plant-based meaty crumbles instead—remembering my reservations expressed previously.

4. Check out the full recipe in Chapter 26.

Taco Guts

I call this taco guts because you decide what goes in your taco. Here are my four favorite options.

1. **Veggie Ground** This is my go-to for taco guts. It's packed with veggies and gets its meaty texture from mushrooms and walnuts. Head to YouTube to find the recipe from Javant at Healthy Vegan Eating. He has hundreds of other delicious, whole plant foods recipes that I know you will love. You can find him at youtube.com/@healthyveganeating

2. **Kung Pao Taco** - Soak Butler's Soy Curls in equal parts low-sugar hoisin sauce, rice wine vinegar, and low-sodium tamari or soy sauce. If you like spicy food, add sriracha or dried Mexican chilies. After the soy curls soften, cook them in the marinade in a skillet.

3. **Tofu Taco** (Recipe from Dillon at Well Your World) - Grate an entire block of firm tofu and toss with Mexican seasoning like Well Your World's Fiesta Fire or Voodoo Seasoning. Add some onion and garlic powder. Spread on a lined baking sheet and bake until golden. Check it every 5-10 minutes and give it a toss. Add some hot sauce at the end if you like it extra spicy.

4. **Tempeh Taco** - Finely chop half of a red onion finely and sauté in a little veggie stock. Add a teaspoon of chopped garlic (1-2 cloves). Grate or crumble a packet of tempeh. Add your favorite taco seasonings and stir. Add spice to your taste preference.

Cheese!

In Chapter 15, you learned why cheese is one of the most challenging animal products to give up. Dairy-based cheese contains addictive compounds called casomorphins—you are literally addicted to the stuff! So, plant-based cheese was born out of a necessity to scratch an itch. But not all plant-based cheeses are created equal. Indeed, the processed oil-laden store-bought versions should be avoided. But you can whip up your own cheesy substitute in a pinch. Try these simple recipes:

Not Queso

If you dread never having queso again, you will LOVE plant-based cheese sauce. There are so many recipes to choose from. Although delicious, many have cashew nuts as a base and contain substantial saturated fat. My favorite is made from veggies with the special ingredient, nutritional yeast, giving the sauce that cheesy flavor. Find my recipe in Chapter 26, or you can scope out chef Dustin Harder's Cheesiest Cheese Sauce from his awesome cookbook *Epic Vegan!* where he uses sauerkraut juice for extra tang (for real)! There's a link to Dustin's book in the resources section. While you are there, make sure to pick up a copy of his other book, *Epic Vegan, Quick and Easy*.

Tofu Ricotta

Tofu ricotta is a game-changer! You seriously cannot tell the difference between regular ricotta and tofu ricotta. (Okay, that may not be 100% true as I have not eaten regular ricotta for years. But I remember it tasting just like this). Use it in your lasagna (with your lentil Bolognese sauce), fill pasta shells with it, and cover it in Puttanesca sauce baked in the oven, or slather it all over toasted sweet potato slices sprinkled with cinnamon. You will wonder why you never ate ricotta like this before. Did I mention it is packed with protein? Find the recipe in Chapter 26.

Parmesan

You may eventually decide not to slather your pasta with parmesan cheese. But in the meantime, try this simple alternative. Toast some blanched almond flakes until golden (don't burn them!), and then throw them in a food processor with nutritional yeast, onion powder, and garlic powder until crumbly. Ta Da! Parmesan cheese. For exact measurements, head to the recipes in Chapter 26.

> To learn more about the dangers of eating dairy-based cheese, please read Dr. Neal Barnard's book *The Cheese Trap*.

Plant Milk

The most effortless change to make toward a more whole plant foods diet is with your coffee and your cereal. No human being needs animal-based milk. Cow's milk contains hormones, antibiotics and other medications, pus (eww!), and saturated fat—none of which you want or need in your body. There are a zillion (yes, that is an actual number) different varieties of plant-based milk available. Wherever you live, there will surely be a huge selection.

Choosing the right one is simple. Use this formula to find a plant-based milk that is perfect for you:

1. Choose the one with the fewest ingredients: No added sugar, salt, oil, gums, or stabilizers. (Milk fortified with added calcium and other vitamins is okay.)

2. Try it out. If you like it, keep buying it.

3. If you don't like it, go back to point number one and choose a different type or brand.

Not all plant-based milk is sold in the supermarket. One of my favorite brands is available only online. JOI stands for Just One Ingredient. Their cashew milk base contains cashews, their almond milk base contains almonds, and their oat milk base contains, you guessed it, oats. Crazy, right? All you need to do is add water for an endless supply of your favorite plant milk. My trick is to blend them all up together. Mmmmm. To get yours, head to addjoi.com/fabuloushealth for a unique discount code on your purchase.

You can also make your own plant milk from scratch. Soy is a little complex as you must cook the beans first, but making your own oat, cashew, or almond milk is easy peasy. For nuts, soak them overnight, discard the soaking water, and then they are ready to use. Oats do not require soaking. Pop your ingredient of choice in a blender with some filtered water and blend. Strain through a nut milk bag (or a fine mesh muslin, hemp, or cotton cloth). Just remember that homemade plant milk has no preservatives. Ensure your storage jars are sterilized, airtight, and your hands are extra clean. Home-made plant milk will last about three to four days in the fridge. If you love gadgets, you can buy a dedicated plant milk machine.

Workbook

Quiz

Answer True or False

1. Going plant-based means throwing out my family's favorite recipes and starting from scratch.
2. Water or veggie broth are excellent substitutes for oil.
3. My life is over now that I'm not eating cheese!

ANSWERS in Appendix

Journal

Today I learned
_____

Today I feel
_____

I am proud of myself today because
_____

One thing I can improve upon tomorrow is
_____

What is my biggest struggle right now?
_____

Who can I ask to support me with this?
_____

What is my main goal this week?
_____

What does my idea of success look like next week?
_____
_____
_____

What three daily actions can I take to reach that goal?

1. _____
   _____

2. _____
   _____

3. _____
   _____

> **Quick Tip**
>
> Make the transition to plant-based eating as simple as possible. Start with your favorite recipes and make them healthier. Let go of the expectation that they will taste the same. They will be different but still delicious.

CHAPTER 20: Creating Healthy Habits

"At any moment, you are one good choice away from a meaningfully better life." James Clear, Author, Atomic Habits

What's In This Chapter?

Getting healthy, losing weight, and reversing disease is less about achieving goals and more about taking daily action steps to reach those goals. The goal is the result of the action steps. The goal becomes an inevitable consequence of the new healthy habits that you do, day in and day out. In this chapter, I will help you start new habits and keep them going forever so that you will reach any goal you put your mind to. I did not invent these strategies. I have learned them over time.

Make Habits Easy

If I told you to eat a pound of kale every morning for breakfast, I bet you would throw this book in the trash right now. Not only would that be completely unappealing, but you might also not know how to prepare the kale or make it tasty. What if I asked you to add a handful of kale to your fruit smoothie each morning? Would that be so hard? What about swapping your cow's milk for plant milk in your morning coffee? Could you do that?

The trick to making a habit stick is to make it a no-brainer. Do you want to exercise every morning? Put out your exercise clothes the night before, then put them on in the morning. Now you are ready to exercise. Just do five minutes. You can commit to five minutes, can't you?

Below are a few habits you can start right now. But beware! Don't start them all. Pick one or two and do them for a month. Use a habit tracker or tick a box on your calendar each time you do the habit. At the end of the month, tally your results.

- Drink a glass of water as soon as you wake up
- Walk the dog straight after breakfast
- Exercise for at least thirty minutes daily
- Choose a healthy meal once per day
- Eat a piece of fruit every day

- Stop scrolling on Instagram an hour before you go to bed

    (write your own)

- _____
- _____
- _____
- _____

Whatever habits you choose, ensure they are the lowest-hanging fruit. What can you realistically do every day? If your first habit is not as easy as brushing your teeth, choose an easier one. Make it personal to you—something you want to do. Then, do it without fail.

Make Habits Replicable

Replicating habits is a skill in itself. You will only repeat a habit if it is enjoyable, helps you reach your goal, and is easy. So, set yourself up for success. What will make you drink a glass of water before breakfast every morning? Do you need a note on the fridge? Do you need to put a glass of water next to the coffee machine the night before? Do you need a reminder alarm on your phone? Whatever you need to make doing the habit inevitable, install a system to make the habit non-negotiable.

Habit Stacking

Habit stacking is where you become proficient at one habit and then use it as a springboard for another. For example, you make a smoothie every morning for breakfast. That's your first habit. Now, put a handful of kale in it. That's the second habit.

You already go to the gym three times per week—the first habit.

You stay fifteen minutes more and get some stretching or meditation—the second habit.

It's just like having a shower and then brushing your teeth. If you do it often enough, it becomes second nature. Stacking habits makes them easier to complete than trying to incorporate new habits by themselves. If you are not already making a smoothie, will you randomly eat a handful of kale? Will you stretch for fifteen minutes if you are not already at the gym? Probably not.

Logging

One of the fastest ways to make a new habit automatic and effortless is to log it. Yes, I know it can be tedious, but it works. There will be no positive change if you refuse to do the work. A habit will not magically manifest itself in your life without repetition. Humans tend to overestimate our good qualities and underestimate our less-than-stellar ones. Did I put that kale in my smoothie yesterday? Maybe, or maybe not. Just tick a box, have a list, and write it down. Log your workouts, walks, the servings of fruit you eat daily, and your water intake. Whatever new habit you want to implement, log it. Then, each week, take a look at your actions. Did you complete the new action each time you wanted to? Or do you see times when you skipped it? Without logging, your brain will trick you into thinking you were perfectly compliant.

The information you gain from logging habits is not meant to point out your failures; it is purely to give you data. Did you go to the gym one time last week instead of three? Think about why. What got in the way? Perhaps three times per week is too much for your busy schedule. Change your expectations. Twice per week might be more realistic for you.

Rewards for Behavior Change

Have you lost weight in the past, and as a reward for being 'good,' you bought yourself a donut or a double cheeseburger? This kind of food reward sabotages your efforts and tells your brain that you are incapable of making healthy choices. Unhealthy food rewards are counterproductive to promoting a healthy lifestyle. Instead, think of longer-lasting rewards that will remind you of your efforts and incentivize you to strive for better health.

A few examples:

1. Buy a new pair of pants in a smaller size than before. Make sure they fit you when you buy them. Don't buy a size too small and hope they will fit later. You want to wear them with pride. If you are worried that you will shrink out of them too fast, that's okay. Pick them up for a bargain at a consignment store or resale outlet. Then, you can sell them back to the store when you need a smaller size.

2. Take an outing to a place you have always wanted to visit but never did. I've lived in Dallas, Texas for over six years and still haven't seen the Dallas Arboretum. There must be hidden treasures in your hometown, too. Make sure you take photos to reflect on the day fondly.

3. Get a new kitchen gadget. Have you been eyeing that Breville air fryer but balked due to the cost? Save those pennies and splurge once you reach a significant milestone.

Milestones don't have to be far off in the future. "When I lose ten pounds" seems so far away. How about rewarding yourself for exercising more than three times this week with a relaxing bubble bath? If you have a day where your nutrition is on point, give yourself twenty minutes to journal your feelings. Whatever makes you feel good, a pat on the back for healthy choices will motivate you to continue another day.

> If you want to learn more about creating healthy habits that stick, I highly recommend James Clear's book *Atomic Habits*. There's a link to it in the resources section.

Workbook

Quiz

Answer True or False

1. The best way to adopt a new habit is to pick the easiest thing first.
2. Habit stacking is where you add a new habit to an existing habit.
3. When you lose weight, the best reward is a massive donut, as the sugar resets your metabolism.

ANSWERS in Appendix

Journal

Today I learned
_____

Today I feel
_____

I am proud of myself today because
_____

One thing I can improve upon tomorrow is
_____

What is my biggest struggle right now?
_____

Who can I ask to support me with this?
_____

What is my main goal this week?
_____

What does my idea of success look like next week?
_____
_____
_____

What three daily actions can I take to reach that goal?

1. _____
   _____

2. _____
   _____

3. _____
   _____

Quick Tip

Don't try to change everything at once. Start a new action and wait for it to become a habit before starting another one.

CHAPTER 21: Putting It All Together

"The choice of diet can influence your long-term health prospects more than any other action you might take."
C. Everett Koop, Former Surgeon General.

What's In This Chapter?

This is my favorite chapter because after reading this far, you will finally put all this newly acquired knowledge into practice. You have learned so much and come so far. Now, it's your turn to make this plan work for you. In this chapter, you will learn three simple steps that will remove all the fear and guesswork of transitioning to a whole plant foods diet to improve your health. Are you ready? Let's go.

Three Easy Steps To Transitioning To A Whole Plant Foods Diet.

Step 1: Start With What You Already Like

Nobody is asking you to drink a kale smoothie every morning (unless you love kale smoothies). This is your life and your journey. You call the shots. You make the best choices for you. No rush. Go at your pace.

The quickest way to start is to go back to Chapter 10 and look at the list of healthy foods. Get out your highlighter and highlight all the foods on the list you already like. Then, think about what recipes you already make that include those foods. You can also head to the back of the book and find a recipe with the foods you already like. Give it a go. Send me a message and tell me how it went.

If you feel stuck, head to the internet and search for recipes with ingredients on your 'already like' list. But before you go down that rabbit hole, try this: Take your favorite ingredients, throw them in a bowl, and eat them—no recipe needed. You might be surprised at how yummy they taste.

Step 2: Swap It Out

Swapping out animal-based foods for plant-based foods is another easy way to make the recipes you know and love with a healthier twist. If you are not sure what to swap for meat or dairy, flip back to Chapter 10 again and see the list of swaps.

Step 3: Try New Things

One of my husband's favorite sayings is, "We don't like new things." Of course, he's joking! But he does love saying it whenever I try a new recipe that includes kale! Sometimes, you will like the new foods and recipes you try, but other times, not so much. Don't throw out the whole plan just because you try something new that you don't like. I've yet to meet an okra I like, but it doesn't stop me from trying new vegetables. It might not be the food, but the way it is prepared. Boiled Brussels sprouts are a bit dull, but air fry them and top them with oil-free kung pao sauce, and they are amazing! Kick fear to the curb and try new things.

Don't go overboard at the Asian grocer and come home with ten new weird and wonderful vegetables. Pick one and find a recipe or cooking method that you think you will like. What's the worst that will happen? Maybe it will cost you a few dollars, and you'll have more food for your worm farm. Or maybe you'll find something sensational that goes into your regular meal rotation. Recently, I grew kohlrabi in my garden. It was a hit! It's delicious, raw or cooked. Step out of your comfort zone and try new things.

The 100% Rule

I considered removing this section from the book because it might scare people off. But once I explain how it works, you'll agree that this rule is awesome! It has taken me years to understand and implement this rule in my life. Now that I have, my life has changed.

Well, what does it mean?

It means that doing something all the time is easier and less stressful than doing it some of the time. For example, if you eat whole plant foods meals all week and then fall off the wagon on the weekends, it has a domino effect.

1. You find it difficult to get back on track and may lapse entirely and give up on your health.
2. You are still eating foods that don't serve your health goals, so you lose momentum.
3. You are still fueling your addiction.

Going all in 100% and committing to the process removes the pressure. There are no cheat days. No hall passes. Just be confident that you are doing your best for your body. Here's an example:

I am an ethical vegan. My moral code tells me I cannot eat an animal. So, if you put a steak in front of me, it is very easy for me to say "No thanks" and not eat it. It's offensive to me. One hundred percent of the time, I will say no to steak, bacon, chicken, dairy, cheese, or any other animal product.

It's not a choice; it's just the way I am.

Corn chips and salsa? Well, that's another story. They have an emotional pull. They are mischievous and devious little snacks. I love the salty crunchiness of the chip mixed with the cool but spicy salsa. Yummy, yummy.

I also know that corn chips and salsa are a trigger food for me. I open the pack, and before you know it, the whole bag is gone! Two thousand calories (most of it oil) in my belly.

Then, my mind starts to waver. I've eaten the chips, so I might as well have a drink and some dessert…Uh ohhhh!

This is where the 100% rule works best.

The trick is to stop these little salty rascals from having any power over me. They do not serve me. They are wolves in sheep's clothing. They pretend to be my friend; instead, they are my enemy, my nemesis.

So, in a moment of calm, I have acknowledged that these franken-foods are addictive and they do nothing for my health. There is no place for them in my life. Period. They are dead to me. So, I broke up with them. Now, I just do not eat them. Ever. It's the 100% rule.

How do you do that? How do you take a food you LOVE and just flat out stop eating it? You have to BELIEVE that it is poison for your body.

Store-bought chocolate cake – poison

Fast food fries – poison

Sugary sodas – poison

Store-bought cinnamon buns – poison

Candy bars — poison

If I told you that in every cinnamon bun, there was a gram of fentanyl* and it might kill you, would you eat it anyway? Hopefully not.

*Disclaimer—Cinnamon buns do not contain fentanyl. I was using this to illustrate a point.

Those 'foods' do not help your health. Those 'foods' only make you happy for the milliseconds in your mouth; afterward, they play havoc with your health. You might not feel it immediately (or you might get bloated and uncomfortable right away), but food devoid of nutrients and high in energy damages your body with every bite.

Set yourself free by kicking them out of your life altogether. Don't grieve for them. Don't pine for them. Say "Good riddance" to those so-called foods that HARM your body.

You have probably thrown your book across the room at this point.

I hear you.

I was YOU.

Until one day, I looked in the mirror naked. None of my clothes fit me. Even my fat clothes didn't fit. I was sluggish; my hair was falling out, my nails were breaking, I had eczema, and I couldn't sleep. I had fat rolls over my belly, hips, and back. I was disgusted with myself.

So, I did a food audit. What was I doing that was making me gain so much weight?

Store-bought cakes – yep

Alcohol – yep

Handfuls of nuts every time I walked past the pantry – yep

Vegan burgers and fries – yep

Processed supermarket cookies – yep

Store-bought hummus and white flour crackers — yes

Corn chips and salsa – oh yeah!

If this stuff puts on the weight, surely not eating it would help me release the fat? It made sense to me. It worked and kept working because those foods no longer tempt me. They don't love me; I LOVE ME! And I love myself with thick hair and clear skin, a full night's sleep, and skinny jeans. I want you to LOVE YOU too. I know you can do this.

Pick one food you know is not your friend and break up with it. You should fill the void with a healthy version of the same food. I didn't give up corn chips. I now make my own corn chips from corn tortillas that I throw in the air fryer for three minutes. They're just as yummy but without the addiction.

When you decide that one food has no power over you and swap it for a healthy alternative, don't stop there. Pick another. Then another and another. Before you know it, no food will have power over you. You will be eating for your health.

Your Ex List

Write a list of foods you eat weekly that do not serve you. Really think about it. Then break up with them. Make a conscious decision that they are poison to your body and they add no value to your life. Then, say goodbye once and for all.

Here are some of mine. Add yours to the list:

1. Cake
2. Corn chips
3. Store-bought vegan yogurt
4. Store-bought granola
5. French fries
6. Champagne
7. Nuts in excess
8. Store-bought hummus
9. Candy bars
10. _____
11. _____
12. _____
13. _____
14. _____
15. _____

I can hear you grumbling as I write this. "There is no way I'm giving up my (insert food here). This woman is crazy."

This is where swaps come in. I don't want to live my entire life without crunchy corn chips and salsa, cookies, or fries. You don't have to either. All you need to do is make healthy versions of these foods and eat them until your heart (and tummy) is content. Score!

There is no missing out, and no willpower is needed to stay on track. That's what 'having your cake and eating it too' is all about.

Head over to the recipes in Chapter 26 for fabulous, healthy versions of your favorite foods, and then cook up a storm. I'd love to hear about the swaps you have made, too. Share your recipes in the online community so we can all try them.

Here are a few swaps that I have made:

Cake

Cake, even vegan cake, is usually made with white flour, white sugar, palm oil, or vegetable shortening. Find a recipe where the flour is whole grain, the sugar is swapped for dates, and the fat is swapped for nuts or avocados. You can even sub out the fat component for beans (more protein) or sweet potatoes (more fiber) in some recipes. But remember, even healthy cake is still calorie dense. Keep the cake for special occasions if you are still trying to lose weight. For yummy whole pant food cake recipes scope out Chef AJ's book *Sweet Indulgence*. There's a link in the resources.

Fries

I already told you about my corn chip hack. I also do this with potatoes to make air fries. The best air fries are pre-cooked and chilled first. Pop your whole potatoes in the Instant Pot for twenty minutes and refrigerate when done. The next day, slice them into fries or wedges and throw them in the air fryer. If you are feeling spicy, toss them with your favorite seasonings. Yummy.

Granola

Despite what food manufacturers would have you believe, most store-bought granolas are not health foods. Granola usually has a ton of added oil and sugar. Head to Chapter 26 and find the best (and healthiest) granola recipe on the planet. Big kudos to Dr Joel Fuhrman for inspiring this recipe.

Yogurt and Hummus

Store-bought plant-based yogurts are full of gums, stabilizers, and fat. You can make your own with one ingredient—soy milk. Head to Chapter 26 to find out how. Store-bought hummus is full of oil. You don't need oil in your life. Homemade oil-free hummus is equally as delicious and costs about half the price of the store-bought stuff. Find out how to make it in Chapter 26.

I could go on, but only you can make the swaps that suit your tastebuds. Think about some of your favorite foods and try to identify the ingredients that make them unhealthy. Then, systematically determine which ingredients you can swap to create a healthier, tastier version. Try making it. You may nail it the first time, or it could taste like cardboard. Don't give up. Keep trying. Use the internet to see how others make it, and keep going until you perfect it to your taste.

No Cheat Days

Don't freak out!!! You are not on a diet. You are changing how you feel about food and choosing foods that align with your health goals. Does that mean you will never again have a donut or a beer? No. Sometimes, you will decide to eat something you know is detrimental to your health. You will make that choice consciously without guilt. Then, your next meal will be healthy food that improves your health. There are no cheat days. You don't have a free pass every Saturday to go to the all-you-can-eat BBQ buffet. Doing that will thwart your efforts, making you more likely to fall off the wagon altogether.

Cheat days originated from the body-building community. Cycling calories and macronutrients inside a structured nutrition and resistance training program can be beneficial. However, I'm guessing you are not training for the Mr/Ms America title, so cheat days are not included in this program. Just eat as much healthy food as you like, and live your life knowing that you are getting the best nutrition for your body.

Progress Versus Perfection

You may think from the last couple of paragraphs that you must always be perfect. That is simply not true. Everyone has their own journey. The most important thing is to do the best that you can do in any given situation. If you are just starting and don't know the difference between arugula and rocket (that's a trick—they are the same thing!), just take a deep breath and start from where you are. Go back a few pages and read 'Three Easy Steps to Transition to a Whole Plant Foods Diet' again, and put them on repeat. Whether that means having a meatless Monday or having a baked potato instead of fries, whatever your starting point is, do your best to make healthy decisions with every meal.

You don't have to get it right all the time. Indeed, if you eat 100% whole plant foods without slip-ups, you will see quicker, more pronounced results. Start where you are comfortable, and push that comfort zone every meal. This does not mean you have to eat foods you don't like. Just add more fruit and veggies. Eat less processed foods. Stop buying meat and dairy. Whatever the next step is for you, take it. If tomorrow you eat more plants than yesterday, you are doing great.

For context, I was a vegetarian for over 30 years before I stopped eating dairy and eggs. Please don't take 30 years like I did. At the time I thought I was doing the best for my body, until I studied the science. Once I learned the truth I went vegan overnight. You have all the information you need now to make the change. Science is evolving constantly, and so will you as new evidence emerges. Try to ditch the foods that harm you, and start by adding as many healing foods to your diet as you can. It's not about being perfect.

It's about being healthier than yesterday.

Sometimes, the options available will be limited and unappetizing. Whenever I go to a Texas Rangers baseball game, as with most sports arenas, the healthy food options are limited. Hot dogs, burgers, fries, and chicken tenders are the norm. But thank goodness the Texas Rangers care about plant-based eaters, as they have a vegan food concession stand. I get myself a salad, whilst Hubs gets a plant-based burger. Is it the best salad I've ever eaten? No. But it's better than nothing. Is the plant-based burger a better option than the beef burger? Absolutely. It is still a processed food, but at least it's not meat. At the baseball game, I make the best choice available. I also go to the basketball and the football. I know what's available at the stadiums, so I usually eat at home beforehand so I'm not hungry at the game. But sometimes that is not possible, so I do my best. Remember this: Every food decision you make can take you closer to your goal or further away from it.

Every Bite Is Helping or Hurting You

Think about that. Every bite either helps or hinders your journey to optimal health. My type-A personality can sometimes make my thinking a little black-and-white, but when it comes to nutrition, it's a strength. No matter how small, every bite we take moves us closer to health or further away. These tiny, seemingly insignificant choices ultimately shape our overall well-being.

Let's take the humble potato, for example. Potatoes are one of the most satiating foods available. They are packed with fiber and energy-giving carbohydrates. They are high in B vitamins, calcium, and potassium. Based on this information, would you agree that eating a baked potato will help you on your health journey? If you agreed, you would be spot on. But slathering the potato in bacon bits, cheese, and sour cream will hinder your health efforts, almost negating the goodness of the potato itself. As does deep frying, mashing with butter and cream, or baking your potato au gratin, slathered with cheese. I'm not saying that you can't eat baked potatoes or fries. But the preparation method, the sauces, condiments, and toppings you use all make a massive difference to the meal's health.

Instead, top your baked potato with homemade chili beans, pico de gallo, tempeh crumbles, and a splash of lime juice! Mmm mmm. Now, you have a healthy, satisfying, and delicious meal. You don't have to count the calories, fat grams, or macros. All you need to do is get that yummy thing in your mouth!

Workbook

Quiz

Answer True or False

1. The 100% rule means you follow the program 100% of the time because it's easier than following it 90% of the time.
2. The 100% rule means you must be perfect for every meal.
3. Making the healthiest choice in any situation will bring you closer to your health goals.

ANSWERS in Appendix

Journal

Today I learned
___

Today I feel
___

I am proud of myself today because
___

One thing I can improve upon tomorrow is
___

What is my biggest struggle right now?
___

Who can I ask to support me with this?
___

What is my main goal this week?
___

What does my idea of success look like next week?
___
___

What three daily actions can I take to reach that goal?

1._____

_____

2._____

_____

3._____

_____

> **Quick Tip**
>
> Cheat days don't help you reach your goals. Sometimes, you will choose your food wisely; other times, not so much. Don't beat yourself up. Just get back to healthy eating with the next bite.

CHAPTER 22: Tackling Self-Doubt

"We gain strength, and courage, and confidence by each experience in which we really stop to look fear in the face... we must do that which we think we cannot." Eleanor Roosevelt

What's In This Chapter?

This chapter offers strategies to keep you on track. Straying off the path and losing sight of your goals can be very easy. When that happens, come back to this chapter for a pep talk. You can do it! I have faith in you.

Have Faith

There is so much dietary advice on the internet it is easy to get caught up and confused. Many of us spend time chasing shiny objects. We jump from program to program, hoping this will be *the one*. After all my years of nutrition education and research, I can confidently say that this way of eating is the healthiest for the human body. Humans are built to eat whole plant foods. It's evidenced by our teeth, the way our jaw moves, and our digestive system. It's also evident by the many different plant-based compounds the human body uses for its metabolism. Quite frankly, if we didn't eat plants, we would die.

The food system, controlled by a few multi billion-dollar multinational companies, has no interest in your health. They only care about profits. This is fine if you have shares in these companies, but it is not great for the common good of humanity. Mother nature provides us with everything we need to be healthy, thriving human beings. Over the ages, people have learned to cultivate plants to our taste preferences and farm them for mass consumption. We learned to cook. But even with farming and cooking, whole plants still have the most nutrition for the human body. No animal or processed food contains as much fiber, vitamins, minerals, and life-giving water as whole plant foods.

Irrefutable scientific evidence spanning half a century from across the globe shows the health benefits of a whole plant foods diet. Tens of thousands of studies all pointing to the consumption of added vegetables, fruit, legumes, and whole grains can't be wrong. So don't sweat the small stuff. Your friends and family—most of whom probably get their nutrition knowledge from TikTok—may want to give you their two cents of advice. Don't be swayed by the opinions of people who have not read the science.

Rest assured that if you stay the course and consistently eat a whole plant foods diet, your health will be in good hands.

There is a caveat to all of this. Nutrition alone is not a cure-all for perfect health. For some, simply changing their nutrition may have amazing health consequences. The reversal of obesity, diabetes, and heart disease can all be achieved through plant-focused nutrition. But only you and your physician know your specific situation. Maybe you still need to be on cholesterol meds, but your angina goes away, and you no longer need a quadruple bypass. I'd consider that an enormous win. Perhaps you lost 40 pounds, but you were hoping to lose 60 pounds. Remember, every pound you lose that moves you toward a healthy weight is doing amazing things inside your body that you don't see.

Be Kind To Yourself If You Slip Up

Everyone slips up—even me. But afterward, you have a choice. What do you do next? Do you throw in the towel and order a dozen wings and a six-pack of beer? Do you stand in front of the mirror and berate yourself for how useless you are? Or do you stop and think about what happened when you slipped up and what you can do next time to make a different choice? What were the circumstances? Where were you? Who were you with? What emotional state were you in? What was going on around you? What were other people doing? All these things play a role in your food choices.

Picture this: *You've had a terrible week at work. Your computer died, and you lost all the work you had been doing for a presentation that needed to be finished yesterday. You tripped and broke your watch on the way to talk to the boss. When you got to your boss, she had her own issues and let them out on you. You were almost in tears. Your workmates offered to take you out after work to make you feel better. They ordered you a margarita to calm you down. Chips and salsa arrived, followed by deep-fried taquitos and quesadillas slathered in sour cream—and that was just for starters. Without thinking about the food, you mindlessly shoved these things into your mouth as you talked about the worst week you've ever had at work. Your sympathetic friends buy you another margarita. You start to feel better. But when you get home, you realize you are not only drunk, but you scoffed 3000 calories that were not on your plan.*

Before you berate your lack of willpower, STOP! It's done. It's over. You can't go back and un-eat those deep-fried taquitos. It doesn't matter. The best thing to do now is think about all the triggers that brought you to that restaurant in the first place.

How did you react when your computer died? Were you distracted, so you tripped and broke your watch? What attitude did you have when you walked into your boss' office? How did you react to her emotional outburst?

All these things led you to going to the bar with your workmates and seeing your healthy plans go out the window. Food—particularly fatty, crunchy, salty food—and alcohol do make us feel better at the very moment we are eating or drinking. There is pleasure in food and alcohol. When you are feeling emotionally bruised and battered, your body's first response is to seek pleasure to make the pain go away. This is normal.

Later, when you logically and calmly see all the many triggers that brought you to that situation, it is much easier to avoid a blowout in the future. A lack of willpower didn't make you eat those extra calories. It was your body not wanting to be in pain.

So, how do we stop this from happening? It takes practice. Like a new habit, you must be aware of what's happening. Think about the times that you have had blowouts in the past. Think about the situation and fill in the blanks below:

Where was I?
_____

Who was I with?
_____

What was happening at the time?.
_____
_____

What emotional state was I in?
_____
_____

How did I feel about my ability to self-regulate?
_____
_____

What actions can I take next time to ensure this pattern is not repeated?
_____
_____

Think about your answers. Is there a pattern?

Do you always have good intentions when you go to your mum's house, but she pushes food on you?

Do your friends buy you alcoholic drinks without asking?

Does your hand subconsciously go into the chip bowl at the Mexican restaurant?

Identify the triggers for you and create a plan to nip them in the bud before they become a problem.

Instead of accepting unhealthy food from your mum, instead, bring healthy cookies to her house and share them with her. That way, both of you get to eat yummy healthy cookies.

Instead of saying yes to that drink, tell your friends in advance that you are trying a dry month and that you'll only be drinking soda water, and lime. No friend would buy someone alcohol if they knew they were trying to get sober.

Instead of diving into the chip bowl at the Mexican restaurant, push them out of reach or send them back before you have a chance to eat them.

Tiny, preconceived strategies for any situation can avert a blowout later down the road. But when it happens, be kind to yourself. Beating yourself up only makes you feel worse and is detrimental to your mental health. Acknowledge it, then make a plan so it doesn't happen again next time. It does take practice, but soon, you'll have the confidence to fly through difficult situations easily.

Measure More Than Scale Weight

The scale is a liar. The scale measures mass—how much your body weighs relative to the Earth's gravitational pull. This should not be your number one metric of success. You are generally weighed with your clothes and shoes at the doctor's office. These items also have a relationship with gravity. Do your clothes and shoes have anything to do with your health? Nope.

Here are a few things the scale does not measure:

- Hydration level
- Fat mass
- Muscle mass
- Bone density/mass
- Waist circumference
- Hip circumference
- Visceral fat
- Subcutaneous fat
- Metabolic adaptations
- Gut microbiota
- Mitochondrial density
- Endurance
- Strength
- Flexibility
- Mobility
- Stress level
- Glucose regulation
- Plaque formation
- Sleep quality
- Mental wellbeing
- Pain level
- Effort
- Habits
- Confidence
- VO2Max—how much oxygen your body can use

I could go on forever because every one of the benefits above (and more) is positively affected when you are adequately nourished with whole plant foods. It doesn't matter if you aren't sure about some of those things; many great things are happening inside your body that the scale does not measure.

Here are a few ways you can monitor your progress:

- How many individual plants did you eat this week? Aim for over thirty—although I bet you can get over fifty.
- How do your clothes and belts fit? Are they looser? Do you need to buy smaller clothes?
- How much energy do you have? Have you stopped your afternoon nana nap?
- How stressed do you get? Can you let go of things you would have been upset about before?
- How many hours of sleep are you getting? Do you fall asleep more easily?
- Can you touch your toes when you couldn't before?
- Can you run for the bus without getting winded?
- Can you climb the stairs carrying a heavy suitcase?
- Are you calmer? More agreeable?
- Are you now a morning person?
- Are you more focused and more productive?
- Have you reduced your over-the-counter NSAID pain medications?
- Is your skin clearer?

When you shift from processed foods to whole, plant-based nutrition, you can expect these benefits and many more. I encourage you to keep a journal to truly appreciate the positive changes. Record every improvement you notice, no matter how small. When you need a reminder of how well this approach is working, revisit your journal. Seeing your progress documented will reinforce your motivation and encourage you to continue on your path to better health.

Fill in the space below: Fabulous things I've noticed about my body since eating a whole plant foods diet:

_____

_____

_____

_____

Self Educate

Nothing tackles self-doubt more than proof that this way of eating has worked for someone else. It can work for you, too. You are so fortunate to have found this way of eating now, as a vast array of books, movies, and websites can help solidify your resolve to be healthy and support you on your journey.

In this book, I've asked you to trust me. Yes, I've provided scientific references for you to check, but nothing is better than self-education. Don't just take my word for it. Explore the world of plant-based science in a way that is relevant to you. If you have heart disease, check out books from Dr. Dean Ornish and Dr. Caldwell Esselstyn. If you have gut issues, look up Dr. Will Bulsiewicz. For PCOS, read Dr. Nitu Bajekal. For diabetes, search Dr. Cyrus Khambatta. Dr. Shireen Kassam is one of the world's foremost cancer and plant foods nutrition experts. There are too many fantastic health professionals to list here, all intent on helping you live a healthy life free of disease.

Use this book as an introduction to whole plant foods nutrition to improve your health and live a life of vitality. These experienced doctors are experts in their specialties. Find them and increase your knowledge of the benefits of whole plant food nutrition to your specific issues.

If reading is not your jam, get the audiobooks or watch a movie. Just search plant-based movies', and open your world to documentaries that will change your life. Here are a few of my favorites:

- Eating You Alive
- Plant Pure Nation
- What the Health
- The Need To Grow

Head to my website, fabuloushealth.net, for links to the movies and more.

Workbook

Quiz

Answer True or False

1. There is no such thing as willpower. When you plan for a situation, food no longer controls you.
2. If you slip up, you might as well go back to your old way of eating.
3. You are not an island. Peel back the curtains and find a community of people on the same healthy path as you.

ANSWERS in Appendix

Journal

Today I learned
___

Today I feel
___

I am proud of myself today because
___

One thing I can improve upon tomorrow is
___

What is my biggest struggle right now?
___

Who can I ask to support me with this?
___

What is my main goal this week?
___

What does my idea of success look like next week?
___
___
___
___

What three daily actions can I take to reach that goal?

1._____
_____

2._____
_____

3._____
_____

> **Quick Tip**
>
> The road to fabulous health is not a straight line. There will be roadblocks and difficult times, but believe that you can succeed—and you will.

CHAPTER 23: Life In The Real World

"Not I, not anyone else, can travel that road for you. You must travel it for yourself." Walt Whitman

What's In This Chapter?

This chapter will navigate the world outside your home, including travel, parties, and family holidays. You will learn how to handle peer pressure and food pushers. Then, you will learn how to read restaurant menus so you can choose the healthiest options available.

Travel

Going on vacation does not mean you have to throw your health goals out of the window, but it would be short-sighted of me to suggest that you can just carry on as usual. I know you want to try all the pasta when you go to Italy. "When in Rome . . .", as they say.

My travel tip is to stay in an apartment with a kitchen or book a hotel room with a fridge and a microwave. When you can prep your own food, you will eat healthier than if you eat in restaurants for every meal. Even if you can only prepare one meal a day in your accommodation, it's better than none at all. I've been known to bring my blender, Instant Pot, and a cooler full of vegetables on road trips!

If you can stay in an apartment with a full kitchen, try to make as many meals as possible, going out for the occasional special dinner. Head to the local store and stock up on fresh fruit, salad greens, oatmeal, some cans of beans, potatoes, and frozen veggies. Or explore the city and find a farmers' market. Shop with the locals and be introduced to new and exciting foods culturally significant to the area.

What if you are at a holiday resort or overseas and cannot bring food, and the hotel does not let you cook food in your room?

Breakfast

Most hotels supply breakfast. Head for the salad bar and start with a green salad. Yes, you can eat salad for breakfast. Then, see if any vegetables, such as grilled tomatoes, asparagus, and mushrooms, are available. They will undoubtedly be cooked in some oil, but don't stress. It will not harm you to have oil for a couple of days, but avoid the Danish pastries, sausage links, and hash browns. If you are staying at a five-star hotel, do not be afraid to speak with the chef and ask them to make you some steamed vegetables, or grab a bowl of oatmeal with berries. Check if the oatmeal is prepared with water or milk. Most likely, it will be prepared with water. You can add soy milk yourself. You might be able to take a couple of pieces of fruit for snacks later.

Lunch

Great on-the-go options include falafel wraps (ask for no tzatziki) or veggie pizza with no cheese (bonus if you can get a whole grain crust). Any pasta with a vegetable or tomato-based sauce is yummy and filling. My favorite is Puttanesca (make sure to ask for no anchovies). Vegetable and bean soups will fill your stomach, and salads are also a great option. The salad formula from Chapter 18 is not just for home use, you can create your own salad when out too.

Dinner

Going to a plant-based restaurant is the easiest way to eat dinner on vacation. But if none are available, Italian, Ethiopian, Indian, Mediterranean, or Thai restaurants are your best bet. These cuisines generally have dishes that are naturally plant-based. You might need to have a quick conversation with the server, but most restaurants are prepared to cater to their customers' dietary requirements.

Eating at Restaurants

As I mentioned earlier, if you can find a plant-based restaurant, there are usually more options. However, many plant-based restaurants in the USA make dishes that try to mimic meat-based dishes using processed meat alternatives. Many meals come with fries, or the food itself is deep-fried. Even though it's plant-based, it may not be healthy. So my family prefers regular restaurants where we can find one or two vegetarian options that can be altered.

The first culprit is oil. Oil is frequently used in restaurants, so unless you know the chef, assume everything is cooked in oil. Look at the menu and find the vegetarian option first. Is it deep-fried? Does it have cheese as an ingredient? Is it smothered in a dairy-based sauce? If the answer is yes, perhaps you are at the wrong restaurant. See what is left when you remove these things.

One of my favorite restaurants lists vegan tofu lettuce wraps on its menu. The description says: crispy tofu, cashews, ginger, sesame, fresh vegetables, lettuce, and spicy vegan mayo. But the tofu is deep-fried, and they come with deep-fried crouton thingies. So most of the calories in the meal come from oil.

I love a good power bowl. Here is the menu description: marinated tofu, shiitake mushrooms, edamame, fresh vegetables, crisp greens, avocado, cauliflower rice, soft-boiled egg and spicy vegan mayo. Sounds incredible, right? This dish is easily made healthier by removing the egg while retaining all its delicious flavors. Because it contains tofu and edamame, removing the egg will not mean you miss out on essential nutrition. If you are watching your fat intake, remove the avocado or only eat part of it.

A Caesar salad usually includes croutons, cheese, bacon bits, and creamy dressing. Taking these things off leaves you with a bowl of lettuce, for which the restaurant will charge you twenty dollars! Don't fall for that. There's no nutrition in a bowl of sad, pale lettuce. Instead, see if you can add things. Ask the kitchen to add some carrots, bell peppers, radish, beans or tofu.

Italian restaurants always have Pasta Marinara (or red spaghetti, as we Aussies call it). You can make that at home with your eyes closed, so ask the server to get the chef to spruce it up for you with extra roasted vegetables.

I thought French cuisine was out of my reach until I went to a French restaurant for a family gathering. I was not involved in the restaurant choice, so I resigned myself to ordering a green salad and going home to make dinner. I told the server I was vegan and asked politely if anything on the menu was not cooked in butter. To my delight and surprise, the chef created the most delicious meal of side dishes: roast potatoes, green beans with almonds, root vegetables, brown rice, and their famous ratatouille. It was delicious! Was there some oil? Yes, however it was such a lovely gesture, and the food was so good that I accepted it gracefully.

I've also been to a steak restaurant, begrudgingly. Again, I was surprised by a humongous baked potato, grilled corn, and a massive serving of steamed mixed vegetables. You should be able to find something to eat at most restaurants. When in doubt, call ahead and see if the chef can cater to your dietary requirements. You may be surprised at what is available to you. The only exception would be a seafood restaurant where all the dishes contain fish or crustaceans. My advice would be to avoid seafood restaurants entirely.

Parties

Parties are a completely different story. The food at parties is usually sweet, salty, and fatty. You know everything you want to eat at a party will likely be unsuitable. There are fizzy drinks, alcohol, and birthday cake; parties are a minefield of temptation.

There will come a time when you go to a party, and the hotdogs, cupcakes, and bowls of chips will not talk to you. When that happens, you will have reached food freedom. But until that time, you need to be prepared for the temptations a party brings. Here are some tips for enjoying the party and avoiding unhealthy foods and drinks.

1. Focus on the people, not the food. Parties are for catching up with old friends or making new ones. The food is just a sideshow.
2. Ask the host if you can bring a dish. Hosts love it when people bring food to parties; it takes a little pressure off them. Make something yummy, but don't tell anyone it's healthy. Definitely don't label it vegan. Everyone will enjoy it and tell you what a great cook you are.
3. When you are offered a drink, graciously accept. "Thanks so much; I'll take a soda with lime." You need not explain to anyone why you are not drinking alcohol. It's none of their business. Just drink your soda and move on. If you are pressed, just say, "I love lime and soda. It's so refreshing. How's your family?". Deflect the conversation away from what you are eating or drinking.
4. Look for the healthy food. Most parties have at least one token healthy plate of fruit, hummus, and veggie sticks. Scope out the healthy stuff and enjoy it.
5. When you look at the cupcakes, hotdogs, or deep-fried chicken wings, try not to see them as food. Look at them and see sickness and pain. I see dead animals when I look at meat, and it repulses me. When I see ice cream, I see tortured cows having their babies taken away from them. I see breast cancer. It is very easy to resist when you can give the party food an alternative identity that doesn't align with your goals.
6. Eat before you go. Fill yourself up with a delicious, nutritious meal before you leave, and I promise the food on display will not call your name.

Family Holidays

Like parties, family holidays can be a minefield. Not just of tempting treats but an emotional minefield. Family members who insist on pushing their food on you or those who want to argue how much humans need meat to survive. It can be tricky to navigate. For your own sake, tackle your family holidays with as much confidence as you can muster. If your family easily sways you, double down on your resolve. You need to stand up for what you believe. If you genuinely believe that a Thanksgiving or Christmas dinner of turkey, ham, and all the fixings will not help you on your health journey, then you must stick up for yourself. Eat only what you want. Get involved in the food preparation. Make delicious dishes that others can enjoy, but don't make a big deal out of them being healthy. Your health is no one's business but your own.

Dealing with Negative People And Peer Pressure

That said, arguing with people who want a fight is easy. You need to be the bigger person. When you become healthier or lose a few pounds, I guarantee that at least one of your circle will instantly and miraculously obtain a doctorate in nutrition. Just remember this: *Never argue with an idiot* (Mark Twain)—people who know less than you will not be persuaded. Just politely refuse to enter into the conversation. You can do that by deflecting the conversation to other things. "How was your vacation?" "Oh, I love that color on you; where did you get that blouse?" "I hear you are renovating your kitchen; tell me more." You get the idea.

If that doesn't work and you cannot avoid questions, just say, "I'm trying to eat a little healthier, and it's working for me." Then, change the subject. Or, "No thanks, I've already had a whole plateful. I'm stuffed." Remember, you are not trying to force anyone else to eat what you are eating. You are not trying to turn people vegan. All you are doing is minding your business and making healthy choices for yourself.

Community

Change unto itself is hard enough, but doing it alone is even more difficult. Being the only person in your family who is eating healthier is challenging. Especially when you learn what devastation unhealthy food can wreak on your health. I know you wish your partner or kids would jump on the healthy train with you, but they might not be ready. So, rather than go it alone, find your tribe. I have a Facebook group* of people on this journey, the same as you. I'd love for you to join this vibrant community that shares your desire to be as healthy as possible.

Join a Meetup. Download the Meetup app and search for whole-plant foods potluck dinners in your area. These are a great way to meet compassionate people and eat yummy food simultaneously. You might make some new friends and score some delicious recipes.

*To join the Facebook group, see the resources section.

Workbook

Quiz

Answer True or False

1. Your travel days are over. Once you start eating healthy food, you will never be able to travel again.
2. Most restaurants will cater to your dietary preferences if you are polite.
3. Arguing with people about your food choices will only stress everyone involved. The best way to deal with antagonistic people is to deflect the conversation elsewhere

ANSWERS in Appendix

Journal

Today I learned
_____

Today I feel
_____

I am proud of myself today because
_____

One thing I can improve upon tomorrow is
_____

What is my biggest struggle right now?
_____

Who can I ask to support me with this?
_____

What is my main goal this week?
_____

What does my idea of success look like next week?
_____
_____
_____

What three daily actions can I take to reach that goal?

1. _____
   _____
2. _____
   _____
3. _____
   _____

> **Quick Tip**
>
> Be prepared in advance for any social situation. Call the restaurant or bring food to a party. Remember, parties and family occasions are about the people, not the food.

CHAPTER 24: Advanced Techniques

"I've always loved butterflies, because they remind us that it's never too late to transform ourselves." Drew Barrymore

What's in This Chapter?

In this chapter, we investigate strategies for when your weight loss stalls or if you feel like the program is not working as well as it should. We will break down your habits so you can take affirmative action to get back on track.

What to Do When You Plateau

We have all been there. You start a new program, and it's working great until it's not working. Any positive changes that you make to your diet and lifestyle will work for a short time. If you stop drinking alcohol, you might lose a couple of pounds, get better sleep, and have more energy. But then change stops. If you go to the gym every day for a month, you might lose weight for the first two weeks, but after that, nothing.

This is called a plateau. It will likely happen after four weeks and again within the first six months. It's very frustrating and can be the impetus to give up altogether and return to old habits. Weight loss, the metric you will likely track, is not linear, so don't stress. Know that this is your body's natural course toward healing.

When you start eating healthier foods, many wonderful things happen inside your body—most of which you cannot see. Your cells are being fueled with incredible nutrition, phytochemicals are working their magic as anticancer antioxidants, water hydrates every cell in your body, and fiber increases your gut microbiome biodiversity. These are just a few things not reflected with the scales or the tape measure.

If you are eating well, getting good sleep, and moving your body, but the scale is not moving or going up—don't stress. Just keep doing the things. It's working, I promise. After three consistent months of eating this way, go back to your physician for another well-person check-up and be amazed at the changes in your body. Sure, you can wait till six months or longer, but after three months the effect of whole plant foods nutrition will be apparent You might see better cholesterol, lower blood pressure, better glucose metabolism, and lower c-reactive protein—just to name a few biometric markers. Seeing these improvements will be the impetus to continue along this journey, regardless of your pant size.

So, when you plateau, the first thing to do is DON'T PANIC. You are doing everything possible to give your body optimal nutrition. Let's look at what could be stopping you from losing more weight.

Stress, lack of sleep, exercise (too much or too little), hormone imbalance, and emotional and mental health all affect our bodies. The scope of this book does not allow me to go into too much detail, but suffice to say, even though nutrition plays a significant part in your health, it's not the only part. I touched on this in Chapter 3, so if you need a recap, please read the section on the six pillars of health again.

A calorie deficit is the only way a human body can lose weight. We discussed this in great detail in Chapter 10 when you learned about the difference between energy density and nutrient density.

When you switch from a diet high in animal products and processed foods, you will lose weight almost instantly. This is because those foods are high in salt; where there is salt, there is water. So, the first thing you lose is excess water in your cells. Then, as you lower your energy density and up your nutrient density, your body obtains all the nutrients it desires. Gone are the cravings, the sugar highs and lows and the late-night snacking. Removing high-calorie foods and replacing them with lower-calorie whole foods is enough to get your body to access its fat stores. Pretty soon though, your body will reach equilibrium. It may be four weeks or 6 months down the line. Your body loves healthy food, and you are getting healthier on the inside, but the weight loss stops (usually before you want it to).

At this point it's wise to look at the other factors contributing to weight loss plateaus. Stress will knock weight loss on the head. The stress hormone, cortisol, is related to the 'fight or flight' body system known as the sympathetic nervous system. Raised cortisol levels caused by chronic stress can increase your appetite, slow your metabolism, and create insulin resistance [116], leading your body to store more fat. Recognizing the stress factors in your life and taking action steps to mitigate them may be enough to kickstart your weight loss.

Stress is also a significant risk factor for increased blood pressure, which contributes to the development of atherosclerosis and heart disease. For more information on stress, refer to Chapter 4.

Let's assume that you are not under stress, that you are getting great sleep, that your relationships are nurturing, and that you regularly exercise. Let's say that you think you are doing all the right things, but you are not seeing any more changes on the scale. It's time to step it up a notch.

Do a 72-hour food audit. Write down every morsel of food you eat for three days. Make one of those days a weekend day. These days do not need to be consecutive, but they must be typical of what you regularly eat. Did you go out for pizza? Did you make cookies and 'test' a few? Did you snack after dinner? Did you get upset and head to the pantry for some dark chocolate? Even if all the food in your house is whole plant foods, you can still overeat calories by not paying attention.

I'm not going to micro-manage you here. You will know 100% after you write down what you eat, where your Achilles heel lies. For me, it's nibbling while making dinner. Or the 4pm cookie break. One cookie is fine. Five cookies... well...not so much.

I'm not good at freestyle eating, but if I have a plan, I'll stick to it. If you are like me, make sure you have your meals planned and prepped so that when dinner time arrives, you won't be left rummaging through the fridge, feeling uninspired, and giving in to the temptation of take-out.

You need to be your own food police. When you review your 72-hour food intake, be honest with yourself. Identify the source of the extra bites, portions, and tastes and nip them in the bud.

The Ad Libitum Lie

You may have heard plant-based doctors talk about eating ad libitum. Ad libitum comes from Latin and means "according to pleasure." When we eat ad libitum, it means we eat as much as we want, without restriction. There is a recurring theme amongst some well-respected doctors that you can eat ad libitum on a whole plant foods diet and still lose weight. This may be true for some people, but certainly not for me or many of my clients. We have been sold a lie that we can eat as much as we want, and the weight will magically come off. I wish it were true, but the human body has other ideas.

Every person is different. A sedentary post-menopausal woman's metabolism differs from an active pre-menopausal woman or a man. If we were so good at regulating our metabolism, every whole-plant-food eater would be skinny, and we know this is not the case. Skinny should not be the end goal anyway. We are looking for healthy. For some of us, that means carrying a few more pounds of fat than we want.

But how do you know you are eating the right amount, and not too much? Just listen.

The Sigh

The most underrated weight loss tool is listening to your body. Sometimes, when people sit down to a meal, they are so hungry that they shovel it all in so fast that they are unaware of their body's satiety cues. (Or is that just me?) Your body will tell you when you have had enough. The Japanese call it *hara hachi bun me*, which translates to "eat until you're 80% full." You will experience it as an involuntary sigh.

Think about your last meal. A little more than halfway through you will have involuntarily sighed. Listen to that sigh. That is your body telling you *hara hachi bun me* — you have had enough. The trick is to stop eating immediately, even if you haven't eaten your favorite roast potatoes yet. Stop, drink some water and have a conversation with your dinner partner. You are done.

You may ignore the sigh and keep eating till the plate is clean, or until you can't put another bite into your mouth. This practice is not conducive to weight loss or health. Even if you are eating a bowl of kale, stop when your body tells you it has had enough. This is one of the most challenging practices to master but try it with every meal. When you feel the sigh, think about what it is telling you.

You won't be missing out on nutrition. Put your plate aside and eat the rest when you are hungry again.

Intermittent Fasting

There is a large body of literature and self-help books about the benefits of intermittent fasting. Intermittent fasting means to fast purposefully for specific times per day or week. Giving your body time without food has many benefits including better glucose control, lower incidence of cardiovascular disease, improved gut microbiota, improved cognitive function and increased lifespan [117]. Intermittent fasting is not for everyone. It can be an excellent way for men to lose extra body fat. But for women, particularly post-menopausal women, it can increase cortisol levels and prompt our bodies to store additional fat, particularly if we are exercising regularly. People fast anyway between dinner and breakfast. If you have dinner between 6-8 pm and breakfast between 7-9 am, you already fast thirteen hours.

Additionally, if you stopped eating last night's dinner at the *hara hachi bun me* (the sigh), you should be hungry again when breakfast rolls around. By all means, if you are not hungry in the morning and you cannot stomach breakfast, then don't eat it. But please do not starve yourself to get in a long fast. It's not helping you. Journalist and professor Michael Pollen eloquently said in his book *In Defense of Food*, "Eat food. Not too much. Mostly plants." I'm not telling you not to try intermittent fasting. If you want to try it, source credible information from respected researchers and see if it works. However, if it does not fit with your lifestyle, don't bog yourself down in restrictive regimes that lessen your enjoyment of food and interfere with your life.

Juicing Versus Smoothies

Who doesn't love a smoothie? Smoothies and juices can be tasty, portable and a great way to get nutrition into your body with little effort. But they may be thwarting your weight loss efforts. Let's start with juicing.

I juice only occasionally. My go-to juice contains orange, apple, kale, ginger, celery, cucumber, and carrot. Sometimes I'll add some turmeric or beet, but never more fruit. The issue with juicing is that all the fiber is removed. If you are only juicing fruit, the result becomes a liquid of easily digestible sugars. They taste great, but raise your blood sugar very quickly and make you hungry. Mixing in at least the same amount of vegetables will attenuate the blood sugar spike a little, but not as much as keeping the whole food intact. Store-bought juices should be avoided as they can contain added sugars and other ingredients.

Instead of juicing these foods, try blending them with water. This way, you will also benefit from the fiber. This is where smoothies come in. You do not need to put every vegetable in the fridge into your smoothie. Be selective and make a delicious, nutritious, filling breakfast. Here is my go-to smoothie.

Berry-Nana Smoothie (Serves 2)

250ml sugar-free soy milk

250ml water

1 cup frozen strawberries

½ frozen banana

1-2 cups chopped greens (spinach, kale or chard)

1 tbsp ground flax

2 tbsp hemp hearts

50gm oats

Blend and enjoy.

Workbook

Quiz

Answer True or False

1. When plateaus arise, it's essential to look at other aspects of our lifestyle such as sleep and stress as they can have a significant impact on our progress.
2. As long as you eat whole plant foods, you can eat as much as you want and continue to lose weight.
3. When our body has had enough food, it tells you by making you fart.

ANSWERS in Appendix

Journal

Today I learned
_____

Today I feel
_____

I am proud of myself today because
_____

One thing I can improve upon tomorrow is
_____

What is my biggest struggle right now?
_____

Who can I ask to support me with this?
_____

What is my main goal this week?
_____

What does my idea of success look like next week?
_____
_____
_____

What three daily actions can I take to reach that goal?

1. _____
   _____

2. _____
   _____

3. _____
   _____

> **Quick Tip**
>
> You are an individual whose body is constantly changing. What might work for your friend or family member might not work for you, and vice versa. All you need to do is start taking notice. Do more of what moves the needle and less of what moves you backwards.

CHAPTER 25: What's Next?

"There is no such thing as failure. Failure is just life trying to move us in another direction." Oprah Winfrey

What's in This Chapter?

Congratulations! By now, you will be well on your way to regaining your health and living a full life of energy and vitality. This chapter offers suggestions on maintaining momentum so you never have to go on a diet again. It also discusses annual doctor's visits, reducing medications, and menopause.

Yearly Checkups

Are you one of those people who only go to the doctor if your arm is hanging off? Do you shy away from medical professionals? Are you fearful of what the doctors might find? Ignorance is bliss, right? Wrong.

Please do yourself and your family a favor by booking a yearly wellness screening. Health insurance typically covers most costs, so there really is no reason not to. It doesn't hurt and it is generally non-invasive. The most important aspect of regular check-ups is getting to know your primary care physician. When they know you and see you year after year, they notice changes in your health that you might not think are important. Changes that may be early warning signs of potential disease. By catching these, you can take affirmative actions together before conditions develop.

At the yearly checkup, the lab will usually measure biomarkers in your blood for cholesterol, vitamin D and B12 levels, glucose control, and check your liver and thyroid. Depending on your age, they might also suggest screenings for breast, prostate or colon cancer and bone density. When you know your numbers, you can make informed decisions about your health. Your numbers might be fine. But if not, your doctor can work with you to create a personalized care plan. So, even if you feel fit and healthy, please get a yearly wellness check-up.

Reducing Medications

It is not uncommon for people's blood pressure to drop within a few days to a couple of weeks of starting a whole plant foods diet. In case this happens, you need to have your doctor on board so they can reduce your medication. After three months on a whole plant foods diet, many people with diabetes show an improvement in their glucose control (HbA1c) such that their medications can be reduced or even stopped. Your total and LDL cholesterol may reach normal levels when you cease eating dietary cholesterol and significantly reduce your saturated fat intake. Inflammation markers may drop, and rheumatoid arthritis symptoms may be reduced.

Menopause

The world is finally talking about menopause! Hallelujah! Half the population goes through menopause, yet it has remained a mystery to many of us for decades. Women suffer through night sweats, hot flashes, weight gain, brain fog, muscle aches, frozen shoulder, mood swings, and so many more symptoms. For a long time, women were told that's just how it is and to deal with it.

You do not need to just deal with it. I'm not a menopause expert, but I have read a lot of research, and I've learned a few helpful tips for women over forty who are approaching or going through menopause.

1. A whole plant food diet can help relieve vasomotor symptoms such as hot flashes and night sweats [118].
2. Menopausal women need more protein. Make sure to include a high protein source in every meal.
3. Menopausal women need to exercise to maintain muscle mass and reduce bone loss.
4. The best exercise for menopausal women is high-intensity short cardio, such as sprints (running, swimming, or biking) and heavy weightlifting [119].
5. You need rest! Don't wear yourself down by over exercising. Take days off (yes, full days off) to recover.
6. Hormone therapy can be a helpful treatment for women if started within ten years of their last period [120].

> For more information on menopause, I recommend Dr. Nitu Bajekal's book *Finding Me In Menopause*.

Living Your Best Life

When you ditch the animal products and ultra-processed foods and start eating clean whole plant foods, expect your life to improve drastically. No longer will you be poisoning your body with excess saturated fat, stress hormones, medication residues, and chemical additives. Instead, you will be flooding your body with health-giving nutrients, cancer-fighting antioxidants, gut bacteria-loving fiber, and a whole host of phytonutrients to help your body reach optimal health.

Expect to lose weight, be more alert, get better sleep, have better digestion, more energy, and more sharpness of thought. You may finally be able to climb stairs without wheezing or chase your dog around the park without collapsing after two minutes. You may gain confidence in your body and socialize more in your community. I wish all of these things for you and more.

We've reached the end of our journey together, but this is just the beginning of your journey to fabulous health. I sincerely hope you embrace the information within these pages with an open heart and a determined spirit. My deepest wish is that you experience profound and positive changes in your health and well-being, reaping the rewards of nourishing your body with whole, plant foods and cultivating a healthy lifestyle. Congratulations on taking these important steps toward a brighter, healthier future. Thank you from the bottom of my heart for your trust and for allowing me to share this journey with you.

Workbook

Quiz

Answer True or False

1. Yearly check-ups are essential to stay informed about your health.
2. Post-menopausal women need adequate protein to maintain muscle mass and bone density.
3. I am truly honored to have been a part of your journey towards fabulous health. This is a trick question. Of course it's TRUE!

ANSWERS in Appendix

Journal

Today I learned

Today I feel

_____

I am proud of myself today because

_____

One thing I can improve upon tomorrow is

_____

What is my biggest struggle right now?

_____

Who can I ask to support me with this?

_____

What is my main goal this week?

_____

What does my idea of success look like next week?

_____

_____

_____

What three daily actions can I take to reach that goal?

1._____

_____

2._____

_____

3._____

_____

> **Quick Tip**
>
> Help others learn this lifesaving information by leaving a book review on Amazon. To keep in touch, join me at fabuloushealth.net or talk to me at terri@fabuloushealth.net

CHAPTER 26: Recipes

"Everything you see I owe to spaghetti." Sophia Loren

Breakfast

Veggies For Breakfast

Prep Time 1 minute
Cook time 3-5 minutes
Serves 1

The simplest breakfast ever. Just make sure you have all your prepared veggies ready to go in the fridge first (or use frozen ones). Just choose your faves, dump and go. You can either microwave or stir fry in a little vegetable stock. Top with some marinara sauce, balsamic vinegar or chili-lime seasoning.

Granola

Prep Time 15 minutes
Cook time 60—90 minutes
Serves 16+

I have adapted this recipe from Dr Joel Fuhrman's Nutritarian Granola recipe. For the original, head to drfuhrman.com

It is absolutely delicious and contains no oil or added refined sugar. Go easy though, as it is high in calories. This granola works as a great topping for berries and home-made soy yogurt.

Ingredients:

1 banana

1 small cup unsweetened apple sauce

½ cup unsweetened soy milk

1 tbsp cinnamon or pumpkin pie spice

½ tsp vanilla powder or 1tsp vanilla extract

4 cups wholegrain rolled oats (not quick oats)

½ cup chopped walnuts or pecans

½ cup pepitas (shelled pumpkin seeds)

¼ cup sesame seeds

1 cup chopped mixed dried Fruit

Method:

1. Blend together the banana, apple sauce, soy milk, and vanilla.
2. In a large bowl, mix the oats, nuts, seeds and spices (do not add the dried fruit).
3. Add the wet ingredients to the dry and mix till combined.
4. Line 2 baking trays with parchment and spread mixture evenly. Do not press into the tray.
5. Bake at 220-250 °F (105-120 °C) for 30 minutes. You can also use the airfry setting if you have a Breville smart oven (just make sure to lower the temperature or it will burn).
6. Remove trays and toss granola with a spatula. Bake for another 30 minutes.
7. Repeat until the granola is dry and crunchy but not too browned.
8. Let cool. Add the dried fruit.
9. Store in an airtight jar in the pantry. This will last a couple of months (unless you eat it first).

Fruit Salad

Prep Time 5 minutes
Cook time 0 minutes
Serves 1—many

Like veggies for breakfast, this is not really a recipe. Just chop up some fruit and eat it. I buy pre-chopped melons and pineapple from the supermarket and add berries. It takes thirty seconds. This is very low calorie, so you may get hungry in an hour after eating it. To add some calories, top it with home-made soy yogurt and a handful of home-made granola.

Soy Yogurt

Prep Time 5 minutes
Cook time 10- 12 hours
Serves 2-4

The brand of soy milk you use is crucial. Look for an organic soy milk with water and whole soybeans as the only ingredients. Avoid milks with added sugars, emulsifiers, flavors, and thickeners. Milks fortified with calcium are fine as long as they contain nothing else. I use Trader Joe's Organic Soy Beverage. If you can't source that, Edensoy is a good brand too. In Australia, try Vitasoy Protein Plus.

Ingredients:

- 1 quart (liter) soy milk—room temperature
- 3 tbsp organic sugar-free plant-based yogurt
- Or 2 capsules of probiotics

Kitchen Equipment:

Yogurt Maker or Instant Pot

3 x 500ml wide mouth glass jars (such as Ball)—sterilized

Or use the container supplied by the yogurt maker

Method:

1. Make sure your jars are clean. Run them through the dishwasher or boil them in water for a few minutes.
2. Add yogurt or probiotic powder (crack open the capsules) to about ½-⅔ cup of soy milk. Mix well, or shake in a jar.
3. Distribute mixture evenly amongst the three jars, (or the one container) and top with soy milk.
4. Shake or stir well.
5. Place jars in the Instant Pot—set it to yogurt for 11 hours.
6. Fill the tabletop yogurt maker with boiling water. Screw the lid on the mixture container and place it in the water. Leave for 11-12 hours.
7. Remove jars from Instant Pot or yogurt maker and refrigerate.
8. To turn your yogurt into cream cheese, strain chilled yogurt in a yogurt strainer or cheesecloth for 1-3 days.

Scrambled Tofu

Prep Time 10 mins
Cook Time 15 mins
Serves 4

This recipe is my go-to Saturday breakfast. I really like making it because it is a nutritional powerhouse! It consists of protein-packed tofu, nutrient-dense greens, tasty veggies, and yummy spices. You can alter the heat and the extras to suit your own taste.

Ingredients:

- 1 packet firm tofu — drained
- ½ red onion — diced
- 1 tsp vegetable stock powder mixed with ½ cup water
- 2 cloves garlic — minced
- 6-8 button mushrooms (I like Swiss brown)
- ½ red capsicum (bell pepper) — diced
- 2 cups baby spinach or baby kale
- 1 tsp turmeric
- 2 tbsp nutritional yeast
- 1 tsp sriracha — to taste
- 1 tsp mixed dried herbs
- 1/4 cup fresh coriander (cilantro)

Method:

1. Open tofu, pour out water and cut into ½ inch (1cm) slabs.
2. Wrap in paper towel and squish out all the water (or use a tofu press)
3. Mix the stock powder with water and place in a pan
4. Add garlic and vegetables (except greens) and cook till tender (about 5 mins)
5. Squish the tofu through your fingers till it resembles scrambled eggs consistency and add to the veg.
6. Add turmeric and dried herbs
7. Add kale, sriracha and nutritional yeast — and stir.
8. Add more water if necessary - but keep it quite dry.
9. Stir through coriander and serve with pico de gallo and chili-lime seasoning or Tajin.

Green Smoothie

Prep Time 5 minutes
Cook Time 1 minute
Serves 1

Ingredients:

- ½ avocado
- 2 cups mixed greens—spinach, baby kale, Swiss chard
- 1-2 cups coconut water
- 1 frozen banana
- ½ cup frozen mango
- ½ small cucumber
- 1 tbsp flaxmeal
- 1 cup ice

Purple Smoothie

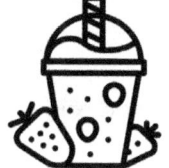

Prep Time 5 minutes
Cook Time 1 minute
Serves 1

Ingredients:

- 1 cup frozen blackberries
- 1 cup mixed greens—spinach, baby kale, Swiss chard
- 1 cup water
- 1 cup unsweetened soy milk
- ½ frozen banana
- 1 tbsp flaxmeal
- Optional—1 scoop of whole food vanilla protein
- 1 cup ice

Method (for both smoothies):

1. Add everything to a blender. Blend for 30-60 seconds
2. Enjoy

Pancakes

Prep Time 10 mins
Cook Time 10 mins
Serves 4

Ingredients:

- 1 cup whole wheat lour (I like einkorn)
- 1 cup soy milk (or plant milk of choice)
- 1 tsp apple cider vinegar
- 1 tsp aluminium free baking powder
- 1 tbsp date powder (optional)
- 1 tsp cinnamon
- 1 cup mixed berries
- 2 bananas
- maple syrup (to serve)

Method:

1. Heat the soy milk for 30 seconds in the microwave to luke warm. Add the apple cider vinegar and set aside to curdle.

2. Sift the flour with the baking soda and date powder.

3. Add the curdled milk and gently mix to combine. Do not overmix. If the batter is too thick, add a little water.

4. Use a cookie scoop to scoop pancakes onto a heated griddle.

5. Cook for 3-5 minutes on each side till golden brown.

6. Slice the bananas lengthways in half and place on griddle with pancakes. Cook till caramelized.

7. Heat the berries in the microwave for a minute. Squish with a fork to make a compote.

8. Serve pancakes with fried banana, berry sauce and some home-made soy yoghurt.

Lunch and Dinner

Basic Pasta Sauce (Marinara)

Prep Time 10 mins
Cook Time 30 mins
Serves 4

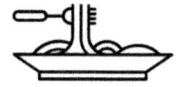

This is an amazingly versatile recipe. You can use it as a base for any kind of tomato-based pasta, bean chili or minestrone soup. Pimp it up, change the herbs and spices and create a whole new dish.

Ingredients:

- ½ red onion—diced
- 1 tbsp garlic—minced
- 1 tsp vegetable stock mixed in ½ cup water
- 1tbsp herbs of choice (I like Italian mix)
- 1 can NAS chopped tomatoes (I like fire roasted)
- 1 can NAS tomato sauce (passata)

*NAS—No added salt

Method:

1. Sauté the onion and garlic in the stock.
2. Add the tomatoes, tomato sauce and herbs.
3. Simmer for 5-10 minutes.
4. Serve over pasta, veggies or baked potato.

Arrabiata

Just add a ton of chili flakes or minced chilis to the basic sauce above to make it *Angry*! Double up the garlic for extra garlicy goodness. Yumm.

Puttanesca

This is my favorite pasta sauce of all time. The flavors explode in your mouth. Keep it spicy or dial it down—whatever you want. Note to those who need to limit their sodium: This sauce contains capers and olives, which are traditionally salty.

Ingredients:

- 1 recipe Arrabiata Pasta Sauce (see above)
- Handful button mushrooms—chopped
- ½ red bell pepper—diced
- 1 tsp capers—chopped and drained
- 1 tbsp kalamata olives—chopped

Method:

1. Prepare as per Basic Pasta Sauce.
2. Add the vegetables to the pan during the sautè stage. Note that the olives and capers will be salty—rinse them to remove most of the salt.
3. Serve with lentil pasta

Minestrone

Prep Time 20 mins
Cook Time 30 mins
Serves 4

This is my favorite soup ever. You can make a big batch and freeze it or eat it every meal for a few days. Delish!

Ingredients:

- 1 recipe Basic Pasta Sauce (see above)
- 4 cups NAS vegetable stock (*NAS—No added salt)
- 1 cup button mushrooms—sliced
- 1 cup carrots—diced
- ½ cup celery—sliced
- 1 cup zucchini—diced
- 1 can NAS canelli (or navy) beans—drained
- ½ cup lentil or chickpea pasta shells
- 1 small handful of fresh basil—chopped

Method:

1. Sauté the vegetables in a little vegetable stock for 3-5 minutes
2. Add all ingredients (except basil) and simmer for 30 minutes
3. Add basil just before serving.

Bean Chili

Prep Time 20 mins
Cook Time 40 mins
Serves 4

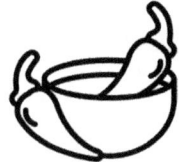

I like my chili spicy, but you don't need to use chili peppers if you don't like hot food. Make it mild or blow your head off—it's your choice. This chili recipe won a chili cookoff in my neighborhood. Nobody even knew it was plant-based.

Kitchen Equipment:

Food processor (optional)

Ingredients:

- 1 recipe Basic Pasta Sauce
- 1 cup soy curls soaked in 1 cup vegetable stock
- 1 can NAS* pinto beans—drained
- 1 can NAS* red kidney beans *(NAS—No added salt)
- 1 cup red bell pepper—diced
- 2 tbsp NAS Mexican seasoning (use in place of the Italian seasoning)
- 1 tbsp sriracha or minced chilis (optional)
- 3-4 sprigs cilantro (corriander)—chopped
- 5-6 pickled jalapeño slices and some juice—diced (optional)

Toppings:

- Cubed avocado
- Pico de gallo
- Chili-lime seasoning (Tajin)
- Shredded cabbage
- Lime juice
- Toasted tortillas

Method:

1. Soak the soy curls in the vegetable stock until soft (I use boiling water to speed things up).
2. Drain soy curls—save the liquid
3. Process soy curls till they resemble crumbles.
4. Cook the pasta sauce as per the recipe above and add the soy curls and all remaining ingredients.
5. Simmer for 30 minutes.
6. Serve with toppings of choice.

Risotto

Prep Time 20 mins
Cook Time 20 mins
Serves 4

Just like basic pasta sauce, risotto can be a base recipe for whatever flavors you desire. Try the classic risotto alla Milanese, pumpkin risotto, spring vegetable risotto or mushroom risotto. Traditional risotto uses arborio rice which is not a whole grain. Try using brown rice, barley or farro for different flavor varieties. Your imagination with risotto is your only limit.

Basic Risotto ingredients:

- 1 ½ cups brown rice—or wholegrain of choice
- 1 onion—minced
- 2 tsp minced garlic
- 1 tbsp mixed Italian dried herbs
- 3-4 sprigs fresh basil
- 4 tbsp nutritional yeast

Variations:

- Milanese—2 pinches saffron, 1-2 tbsp cashew butter
- Pumpkin—roasted pumpkin, toasted almonds
- Mushroom—sautéed mushrooms, green peas, shallots
- Spring vegetable—sugar snap peas, asparagus, broccoli, zucchini

Method:

1. Prepare your flavor ingredients—set aside.

2. Sauté the onion and garlic in a little stock.
3. Add the rice and stir, adding more liquid as the grain absorbs it.
4. Continue to add more liquid as the rice cooks.
5. When the rice is al dente, add the flavor ingredients
6. Serve with fresh basil and a side salad.

Shepherd's Pie

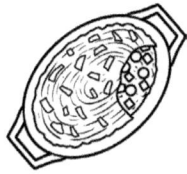

Oven to 350°F (180°C)
Prep Time 20 mins
Cook Time 30-40 mins
Serves 6

The base of this dish can be used for many different recipes. Use it between pasta sheets, and it becomes lasagna. Have it on wholegrain toast for breakfast or an easy lunch. You can even put it in a bun and call it a Sloppy Joe.

Ingredients:

- 2 cans NAS brown lentils (or 1 cup raw soaked and cooked)
- 2 cloves (or more) garlic—crushed
- ½ large onion—minced
- 5-6 cups mixed veggies (mushrooms, zucchini, carrot)—grated or pulverized in the food processor
- 300ml NAS passata (tomato sauce)
- 2 tbsp tomato paste
- 1 tbsp mixed Italian herbs
- 1 cup NAS vegetable stock (*NAS—No added salt)
- 1 Tbsp vegan Worcestershire sauce
- ½ tsp liquid smoke

   Mash Topping

- 2 large potatoes
- ¼ cauliflower
- 2 cups NAS vegetable stock
- 1tsp garlic powder
- 1 tsp onion powder
- 2 tbsp nutritional yeast

DIY Parmesan Cheese

- 2 tbsp nutritional yeast
- 2 tbsp slivered almonds (lightly roasted)
- 1 tsp onion powder
- 1 tsp garlic powder

Method

1. Peel and chop potatoes, floret cauliflower and boil in stock till tender.
2. Drain, add garlic powder, onion powder and nutritional yeast.
3. Mash or mix with an electric beater until fluffy. If needed, use some of the cooking water to loosen. Set aside.
4. Meanwhile: Sauté onion and garlic in a little stock.
5. Add all other ingredients. Simmer for 30 minutes uncovered to soak up most of the liquid.
6. Ladle filling into a Pyrex baking dish.
7. Top with mashed potato and cauliflower mix. Sprinkle on DIY Parmesan
8. Bake for 20-30 mins or until brown on top.

Lasagna

Prep Time 40 mins
Cook Time 30-40 mins
Serves 6

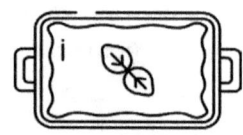

With two easy base recipes and a very simple bechamel cheese sauce, this lasagna is a cinch to whip up. Even on a weeknight.

Kitchen Equipment:

Oven

Blender
9x13 inch Pyrex baking dish

Ingredients:

- 1 batch Shepherds Pie Filling
- ¼ cup NAS tomato sauce
- 1 bag organic baby spinach

- 1 packet whole grain lasagna sheets
- 1 batch DIY parmesan cheese

Cheesy Tofu Bechamel

Ingredients:

- 1 packet silken tofu
- ½ cup soy milk (or plant milk of choice)
- ½ cup nutritional yeast
- Juice of ½ lemon
- 1 tsp miso paste

Method

1. Make the Shepherd's Pie Filling (method above)
2. Soak the lasagna sheets in a single layer in a baking dish filled with hot water to soften.
3. Make the bechemel: Blend the tofu, nutritional yeast, miso and lemon juice. Set aside.
4. Make the Lasagna: Add 2 tbsp tomato sauce to the bottom of a 9x13 Pyrex lasagne dish and event spread to cover.
5. Place 3-4 lasagna sheets in the dish to form a pasta layer.
6. Top with a layer of Shepherd's Pie filling and then a layer of baby spinach.
7. Add another layer of lasagna sheets, Pie filling and spinach.
8. If there is room in the dish, add another layer.
9. Top with a layer of lasagna sheets.
10. Smother the whole dish in cheesy tofu bechamel and top with DIY parmesan.
11. Bake at 350°F (180°C) for 30-40 minutes or until golden brown.
12. Allow to cool for 10 minutes before slicing into 6 portions.
13. Serve with side salad.

Black Bean and Tempeh Casserole

Prep Time 40 mins
Cook Time 15 mins
Serves 4

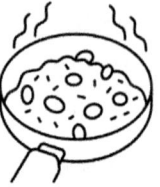

This is an easy dish that will quickly become a staple. Swap out the black beans for any firm-skinned beans you like. Kidney beans or black-eyed peas work equally well.

Ingredients:

- 1 packet tempeh, cubed
- 150g sugar snap peas
- 200g broccoli — cut into florets
- 1 red capsicum (bell pepper) — cubed or sliced
- ½ spanish (red) onion — chopped
- 1 large carrot — sliced
- 1 zucchini — sliced
- 100g button mushrooms — sliced
- 1 can NAS black beans, drained
- 1 corn cob (or ½ cup frozen corn)
- 1 can NAS tomato sauce
- 1 can NAS chopped tomatoes
- Herbs of choice

Tempeh Marinade:

- 2 tbsp liquid aminos (or tamari or low sodium soy sauce)
- 2 tbsp lime juice
- 2 tbsp maple syrup
- 1 tsp minced ginger
- 1 tsp minced garlic
- 1 small minced chili or 1 tsp sriracha
- 1 tbsp liquid smoke

Method:

1. Cut tempeh into small ½ in (1cm) cubes.
2. Mix all marinade ingredients and soak tempeh in marinade for 30 mins.
3. Cook tempeh in an iron skillet till all marinade is absorbed.
4. Stir continuously.
5. At the same time, blacken the corn on a grill, then remove kernels.
6. Add everything (except beans and tempeh) to a wok with a little vegetable stock.
7. Stir fry for 5-10 mins or until cooked to the preferred texture.
8. Add beans and tempeh and cook further 3-4 mins until heated.
9. Serve with quinoa or other grain if desired.

Bean Burgers

Prep Time 10 mins
Cook Time 10 mins
Serves 8

Burgers are one of the most versatile foods to make. You can swap any of the ingredients to suit your taste or occasion. This is more of a formula than a recipe. Make it your own. This works best if you have prepared ingredients. If not, add the cooking time.

Ingredients:

- 1 cup cooked starchy vegetable (potato, sweet potato, yam, pumpkin)
- 1 cup cooked whole grain (brown rice, quinoa, farro, millet)
- 1 cup cooked or canned legumes (lentils, black beans, chickpeas)
- ½ cup whole rolled oats
- 1 cup shredded vegetable (carrot, zucchini, butternut squash)
- 2 or more tbsp herbs and spices of choice (Italian blend, Mexican blend, Indian blend)
- 2 tbsp ground flax mixed with 6 tbsp warm water

Method:
1. Place everything in a large food processor and pulse until combined. If you don't have a food processor, you can mash each ingredient separately and stir together.
2. If the mixture is too wet, add some more oats.

3. Shape into burger sized patties.
4. Cook on a griddle plate for 5 minutes each side or until brown.
5. Can be frozen.

Mike's Butter Beans

Prep Time 10 mins
Cook Time 5 mins
Serves 4

This recipe was first introduced to me by my friend Mike, who probably didn't invent it. It's the world's quickest instant dinner recipe. I hope you will try it.

Ingredients:

- 2 cans NAS butter beans (keep the liquid)
- 1 punnet cherry tomatoes
- 2 huge handfuls of baby spinach
- 1 tbsp apple cider vinegar
- 2 tbsp sun dried tomato paste
- 1-2 tsp roasted garlic puree
- 1 small chili pepper (optional)

Method:

- Put 1½ cans of butter beans (including liquid) in a pan.
- Use a stick blender to puree the remaining 1/2 can of beans. Add to the mixture
- Add everything else and simmer for 5 mins.
- Serve with side salad.

Extras

Cheezy Sauce

Prep Time 10 mins
Cook Time 5 mins
Serves 4

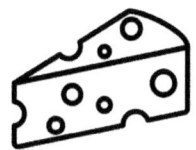

Ingredients:

- 1 carrot
- 1 potato
- ½ a large onion
- 1 tsp garlic, crushed
- 2 cup NAS vegetable stock
- ½ cup raw cashews
- 2 tbsp nutritional yeast
- 1 tsp miso paste
- ½ tsp cayenne pepper or paprika to taste
- 1 tsp apple cider vinegar
- 1 tbsp Dijon mustard
- 1 packet lentil pasta macaroni
- 1 head steamed broccoli to serve (optional)
- pepper to taste
- 3-4 tbsp toasted whole wheat breadcrumbs (optional)

Method:

1. Chop carrot, potato, onion into 2 inch chunks
2. Add veggies, cashews, stock and garlic to a saucepan and simmer till tender.
3. Once the veggies are cooked, transfer them, including the cooking water, to a high speed blender. NOTE: If your blender is not rated for boiling liquids, please wait for the mixture to cool down before blending.
4. Add mustard, spices, nutritional yeast and miso—blend until smooth.
5. Taste and adjust spices as necessary
6. Use immediately or refrigerate for up to 5 days.

Mac'n'Cheeze

1. Pour sauce over cooked pasta and top with steamed broccoli.
2. Place pasta and broccoli in ovenproof dish and top with sauce. Stir to combine.
3. Sprinkle with breadcrumbs.
4. Bake in oven at 350°F (180°C) for 20 minutes or until browned.
5. Serve with green salad.

Tofu Ricotta

Prep Time 5 mins
Cook Time 0 mins
Serves Lots

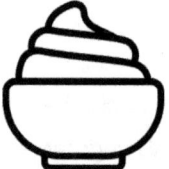

Making lasagna? Stuffed pasta shells? Or maybe you are hankering for some sweet potato toast. This tofu ricotta fits the bill. It's creamy and delicious and you will never miss dairy-based ricotta again.

Ingredients:

- 1 block firm tofu
- 1 tsp miso paste
- 2 tsp lemon juice
- 2-3 tbsp nutritional yeast

Method:

1. Drain the water from the tofu — no need to press.
2. Place into blender with all ingredients.
3. Blend till smooth.
4. Store in a mason jar with an airtight lid for up to 4 days. Or use immediately.

Tofu Mayo

Prep Time 5 mins
Cook Time 0 mins
Serves Lots

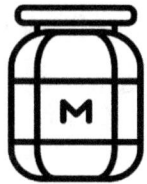

I have a confession to make. I never liked mayonnaise before I found this recipe from Jill McKeever on YouTube. For me, mayo was always gloops of fat and eggs. Yuk! This mayo is a game changer. It's high protein, oil free and delicious! You can also use it as a base to make remoulade and thousand island dressing. For more awesome recipes from Jill, check out her YouTube channel

youtube.com/@JillMcKeever or her website jillmckeever.com.

Thanks very much Jill for allowing me to reprint this recipe.

Ingredients:

- 6-ounces firm tofu
- 1/2 cup water
- 2 tbsp chia seeds
- 2 1/2 tbsp lemon juice
- 2 tbsp apple cider vinegar
- 2 tsp rice vinegar
- 1/2 tsp Dijon mustard
- 1/2 tsp salt (optional)
- 1/2 large pitted date

Method:

- Blend until smooth. Be patient, it takes several minutes to get there.
- Store in an airtight glass jar in the fridge for up to 2 weeks.

Mushroom Gravy

Prep Time 5 mins
Cook Time 10 mins
Serves 4

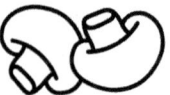

Ingredients:

- 1 punnet brown button mushrooms (sliced)
- 2 tbsp wholemeal flour (or garbanzo bean flour)
- 1/2 red onion (minced)
- 1.5 cups vegetable stock
- 1 tsp Italian seasoning
- 1/2 tsp minced garlic
- 2 tbsp nutritional yeast
- 1 tsp miso paste

Method:

1. Brown the onions, garlic and mushrooms in a saucepan. Splash with a little stock to prevent them from sticking.
2. Add the cooked veggies and all other ingredients to a blender and blend.
3. Return mixture o the pan and cook for 5 minutes to thicken.

Hummus

Prep Time 10 mins
Cook Time 0 mins
Serves Lots

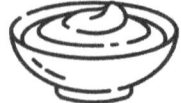

Ingredients:

- 1 can NAS garbanzo beans (chickpeas) — liquid removed but not rinsed. Keep the liquid.
- 2 tbsp tahini
- 1 tsp miso paste
- 2 tbsp lemon juice
- 1 tsp garlic (minced)
- 1/2 tsp Smoked Paprika

Method:

1. Add everything to a blender and blend.
2. Slowly add some of the bean liquid (aquafaba) to reach the desired consistency.
3. Will keep in the refrigerator for up to a week.

Snacks

Oat Cookies

Prep Time 10 mins
Cook Time 15 mins
Serves 24-30

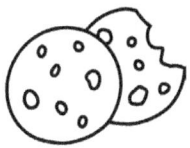

These cookies are my go-to recipe for a healthy afternoon snack with a cup of English Breakfast tea. Recently I pimped them up so that not only are they delicious, but they are also a good source of protein. Keep them on hand in the freezer so you are never without a crunchy snack.

Kitchen equipment:

Food processor or high-speed blender
Oven or toaster oven
Small cookie scoop

Basic Recipe Ingredients:

- 2 ripe bananas
- 1 can NAS garbanzo beans (chickpeas) — liquid removed but not rinsed.
- 2 cups whole rolled oats
- 1 tsp vanilla extract
- 1 tsp cinnamon

Options

The sky is the limit with the variations you can make with these cookies. Here are just a few of my favorite additions. Pick one or two to give you endless flavor combinations:

Vegan chocolate chips
Walnuts
Dried cranberries
Dried cherries

Raisins
Grated ginger
Peanut powder
Dried Apricots

Method:

1. Process the banana till smooth.
2. Add the chickpeas and blend until smooth. You want a little bean juice still on the beans.
3. Add the vanilla and oats. Process until smooth for a smoother cookie. For a chunkier cookie, pulse until combined.
4. Stir in additives (don't blend).
5. Line a baking sheet with baking paper. Use the cookie scoop to form cookie balls. Then use a fork dipped in the bean juice to squash each cookie.
6. Bake at 350°F (180°C) for 13-15 minutes or until brown.
7. Allow to cool and store in an airtight container in the freezer. They will remain crunchy. They will last up to 5 days in the fridge but go soggy.

Tofu Chocolate Mousse

Prep Time 10 mins
Refrigerator Time 30-60 minutes
Serves 4

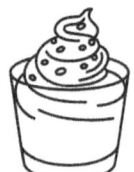

If you are looking for a high-protein snack or dessert, you can't go past tofu chocolate mousse. It satisfies a sweet craving and stops you from reaching for the ice cream.

Ingredients:

- 1 block silken tofu
- 4 tbsp pure cocoa (cacao) powder
- 4 tbsp date powder or 2-3 tbsp maple syrup
- ½ tsp vanilla extract
- 1 shot of espresso (optional)

Method:

1. Blend everything together (make sure your espresso is cold)
2. Separate into four individual serving containers with airtight lids and refrigerate for up to a week.
3. Serve with fresh raspberries and homemade soy yogurt.

Date Snickers

Prep Time 1 min
Cook Time 0 mins
Serves 1

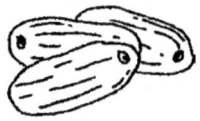

My favorite chocolate bar of all time was the Snickers. I can't recreate the nougat filling, but I can get a sweet caramel, nutty chocolate fix with these 1-minute Snickers wannabes. I urge you to only make one at a time or store them in the freezer if you make more. They are hard to resist.

Ingredients:

- 1 big juicy medjool date
- ½ tsp peanut butter (use PB2 powder for less fat)
- 3-4 mini vegan chocolate Chips
- 3-4 dry-roasted peanuts

Method:

1. Cut the date in half on one side and open it up flat. Take the pit out and discard.
2. Slather on the peanut butter (or PB2)
3. Add a row of chocolate chips and a row of peanuts.
4. Close the two sides back together.
5. Try not to eat it all in one bite!

Chia and Banana Pudding

Prep Time 5 mins
Fridge Time 30—60 mins
Serves 2

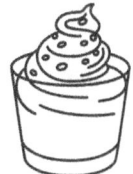

Chia seeds are packed with protein and fiber. When hydrated, they swell nine times their size. Chia pudding has a gelatinous texture that some people love and others hate. I'll let you be the judge.

Ingredients:

- 2 tbsp chia seeds
- 1 cup soy milk
- 1 ripe banana

- ½ tsp ground cinnamon
- ½ tsp vanilla extract
- Handful of blueberries, for topping

Method:

1. Blend everything (except blueberries) until smooth

2. Separate into two servings. Parfait glasses if you are eating them the same day or airtight jars if not.

3. Top with blueberries prior to serving.

Gelato

Prep Time 10 mins
Freeze Time 60 mins plus
Serves — lots

Traditional Italian gelato, like ice cream, is made with milk. Here, we skip the milk and use fruit. Remember to allocate freeze time.

Kitchen equipment:

High speed blender, Yonanas machine, Ninja Creamy or Omega Cold Press Juicer

Ingredients:

- Frozen fruit of choice: banana, mango, strawberry, cantaloupe, cherry etc
- lime juice
- soy milk (optional)
- vanilla (optional)

Method:

1. Using your equipment of choice, blend the fruit till smooth. NOTE: fruit MUST be frozen first.

2. Add a splash soy milk for a creamier gelato (not too much).

3. Or add lime juice to brighten the flavor to taste (but not if you add the soy).

4. Re-freeze for at least 1 hour or use in the Ninja Creamy as per instructions.

Appendix — Quiz Answers

Chapter 3: 1.T, 2.T, 3.F, 4.F

Chapter 4: 1.F, 2.T, 3.T

Chapter 5: 1.F, 2.T, 3.T, 4.F

Chapter 6: 1.Carbohydrate, Protein, Fat, Alcohol, 2.T, 3.F, 4.T

Chapter 7: 1.Animal products, Sugar, Oil, Ultra-Processed foods, Alcohol and Salt, 2. Nine, Seven. 3.F, 4.T, 5.T

Chapter 8: 1.DEXA, 2.0.7, 3.F, 4.F, 5.T, 6.F

Chapter 9: 1.T, 2.T, 3.F, 4.F

Chapter 10: 1.T, 2.T, 3.F, 4.T, 5.T, 6.F

Chapter 11: 1.T, 2.T, 3.F, 4.T

Chapter 12: 1.Animal, 2.90%, 3.No, 4.Animal origin high in fat, 5. Cheese

Chapter 14: 1.F, 2.T, 3.T, 4.T

Chapter 15: 1.F, 2.T, 3.F, 4.T

Chapter 16: 1.F, 2.T, 3.T

Chapter 17: 1.F, 2.T, 3.T

Chapter 18: 1.T, 2.F, 3.F, 4.F

Chapter 19: 1.F, 2.T, 3.F

Chapter 20: 1.T, 2.T, 3.F

Chapter 21: 1.T, 2.F, 3.T

Chapter 22: 1.T, 2.F, 3.T

Chapter 23: 1.F, 2.T, 3.T

Chapter 24: 1.T, 2.F, 3.F

Chapter 25: 1.T, 2.T, 3.T

Bibliography

1. Fraser GE et al, 2020. Dairy, soy, and risk of breast cancer: those confounded milks. Available from: https://doi.org/10.1093/ije/dyaa007

2. Aune D et al, 2015. Dairy products, calcium, and prostate cancer risk: a systematic review and meta-analysis of cohort studies. Available from: https://www.sciencedirect.com/science/article/pii/S0002916523272524

3. Canada Health, 2022. Canada's dietary guidelines. Available from: https://food-guide.canada.ca/en/guidelines/

4. German Society for Nutrition, DGE-Nutrition circle. Available from: http://www.dge.de/gesunde-ernaehrung/gut-essen-und-trinken/dgeernaehrungskreis/

5. Diabetes Prevention Program Research Group, 2002. Reduction in the incidence of type 2 diabetes with lifestyle intervention or metformin. Available from: https://www.ncbi.nlm.nih.gov/pmc/articles/PMC1370926/

6. Naci H et al, 2019. How does exercise treatment compare with antihypertensive medications? A network meta-analysis of 391 randomised controlled trials assessing exercise and medication effects on systolic blood pressure. Available from: https://bjsm.bmj.com/content/53/14/859

7. Noetel M et al, 2024. Effect of exercise for depression: systematic review and network meta-analysis of randomised controlled trials. Available from: https://www.bmj.com/content/384/bmj-2023-075847

8. Harvard Health, 2011. Understanding the stress response. Available from: https://www.health.harvard.edu/staying-healthy/understanding-the-stress-response

9. American Lung association, 2024. Health effects of smoking. Available from: https://www.lung.org/quit-smoking/smoking-facts/health-effects/smoking

10. Leone A, 2012. How and why chemicals from tobacco smoke can induce a rise in blood pressure. Available from: https://wjgnet.com/2220-3192/full/v1/i1/10.htm

11. Cappuccio FP et al, 2008. Meta-analysis of short sleep duration and obesity in children and adults. Available from: https://doi.org/10.1093/sleep/31.5.619

12. Mineo L, 2017. Good genes are nice, but joy is better. Available from: https://news.harvard.edu/gazette/story/2017/04/over-nearly-80-years-harvard-study-has-been-showing-how-to-live-a-healthy-and-happy-life/

13. Livingston G et al, 2020. Dementia prevention, intervention, and care: 2020 report of the Lancet commission. Available from: https://www.thelancet.com/journals/lancet/article/PIIS0140-6736(20)30367-6/fulltext

14. World Health Organization, 2025. Cancer. Available from: https://www.who.int/news-room/fact-sheets/detail/cancer

15. Anand P et al, 2008. Cancer is a preventable disease that requires major lifestyle changes. Available from: https://pubmed.ncbi.nlm.nih.gov/18626751/

16. T. Colin Campbell, 2004. The China Study. Available from: https://nutritionstudies.org/the-china-study/

17. IARC, 2018. Red meat and processed meat. Available from: https://publications.iarc.fr/book-and-report-series/iarc-monographs-on-the-identification-ofcarcinogenic-hazards-to-humans/red-meat-and-processed-meat-2018

18. Cho E et al, 2003. Premenopausal fat intake and risk of breast cancer. Available from: https://academic.oup.com/jnci/article-abstract/95/14/1079/2520334?redirectedFrom=fulltext

19. Penniecook-Sawyers JA et al, 2016. Vegetarian dietary patterns and the risk of breast cancer in a low-risk population. Available from: https://www.ncbi.nlm.nih.gov/pmc/articles/PMC4907539/

20. Orlich MJ et al, 2022. Dairy foods, calcium intakes, and risk of incident prostate cancer in Adventist Health Study–2. Available from: https://www.ncbi.nlm.nih.gov/pmc/articles/PMC9348981/

21. Messina M, 2021. Origins of the soy feminization myth. Available from: https://sniglobal.org/origins-of-the-soy-feminization-myth

22. Messina M et al, 2022. Neither soy foods nor isoflavones warrant classification as endocrine disruptors: a technical review of the observational and clinical data. Available from: https://pubmed.ncbi.nlm.nih.gov/33775173

23. Messina et al, 2022. The health effects of soy: A reference guide for health professionals. Available from: https://www.ncbi.nlm.nih.gov/pmc/articles/PMC9410752

24. Cordova R et al, 2023. Consumption of ultra-processed foods and risk of multimorbidity of cancer and cardiometabolic diseases: a multinational cohort study. Available from: https://www.thelancet.com/journals/lanepe/article/PIIS2666-7762(23)00190-4/fulltext

25. Hastert TA et al, 2013. Adherence to WCRF/AICR cancer prevention recommendations and risk of post-menopausal breast cancer. Available from: https://www.ncbi.nlm.nih.gov/pmc/articles/PMC3774119/

26. Farvid MS et al, 2020. Fiber consumption and breast cancer incidence: A systematic review and meta-analysis of prospective studies. Available from: https://pubmed.ncbi.nlm.nih.gov/32249416/

27. Hu J et al, 2023. Use of dietary fibers in reducing the risk of several cancer types: An umbrella review. Available from: https://www.mdpi.com/2072-6643/15/11/2545

28. Peto R et al, 1981. Can dietary beta-carotene materially reduce human cancer rates? Available from: https://www.nature.com/articles/290201a0

29. Song B et al, 2023. Inhibitory potential of resveratrol in cancer metastasis: from biology to therapy. Available from: https://www.ncbi.nlm.nih.gov/pmc/articles/PMC10216034/

30. Gibellini L et al, 2011. Quercetin and cancer chemoprevention. Available from: https://onlinelibrary.wiley.com/doi/abs/10.1093/ecam/neq053

31. Elkashty OA & Tran SD, 2021. Sulforaphane as a promising natural molecule for cancer prevention and treatment. Available from: https://doi.org/10.1007/s11596-021-2341-2

32. IDF Diabetes Atlas 2025 Available from: https://diabetesatlas.org/resources/idf-diabetes-atlas-2025/

33. Lean ME et al, 2018. Primary care-led weight management for remission of type 2 diabetes (DiRECT): an open-label, cluster-randomised trial. Available from: https://www.sciencedirect.com/science/article/pii/S0140673617331021

34. Kahleova H et al, 2024. Effect of a dietary intervention on insulin requirements and glycemic control in type 1 diabetes: A 12-week randomized clinical trial. Available from: https://doi.org/10.2337/cd230086

35. Li L, 2022. Gestational diabetes, subsequent type 2 diabetes, anfd food security status: National health and nutrition examination survey 2007-2018. Available from: https://www.cdc.gov/pcd/issues/2022/22_0052.htm

36. CDC, 2022. Gestational diabetes. Available from: https://www.cdc.gov/diabetes/basics/gestational.html

37. Ornish D et al, 2024. Effects of intensive lifestyle changes on the progression of mild cognitive impairment or early dementia due to Alzheimer's disease: a randomized, controlled clinical trial. Available from: https://doi.org/10.1186/s13195-024-01482-z

38. Licher S et al, 2019. Genetic predisposition, modifiable risk factor profile and long-term dementia risk in the general population. Available from: https://www.ncbi.nlm.nih.gov/pmc/articles/PMC6739225/

39. Janson J et al, 2004. Increased risk of type 2 diabetes in Alzheimer disease. Available from: https://doi.org/10.2337/diabetes.53.2.474

40. CDC, 2024. About cholesterol. Available from: https://www.cdc.gov/cholesterol/about/index.html

41. Mach F et al, 2020. 2019 ESC/EAS Guidelines for the management of dyslipidaemias: lipid modification to reduce cardiovascular risk: The Task Force for the management of dyslipidaemias of the European Society of Cardiology (ESC) and European Atherosclerosis Society (EAS). Available from: https://doi.org/10.1093/eurheartj/ehz455

42. O'Keefe JH et al, 2004. Optimal low-density lipoprotein is 50 to 70 mg/dl: lower is better and physiologically normal. Available from: https://www.jacc.org/doi/full/10.1016/j.jacc.2004.03.046

43. Ornish D et al, 1990. Can lifestyle changes reverse coronary heart disease? The lifestyle heart trial. Available from: https://pubmed.ncbi.nlm.nih.gov/1973470/

44. Esselstyn CB et al, 2014. A way to reverse CAD? Available from: https://www.mdedge.com/familymedicine/article/83345/cardiology/way-reverse-cad

45. Cuspidi C et al, 2018. Treatment of hypertension: The ESH/ESC guidelines recommendations. Available from: https://www.sciencedirect.com/science/article/pii/S1043661817311179

46. McEvoy JW et al, 2024. 2024 ESC Guidelines for the management of elevated blood pressure and hypertension: Developed by the task force on the management of elevated blood pressure and hypertension of the European Society of Cardiology (ESC) and endorsed by the European Society of Endocrinology (ESE) and the European Stroke Organisation (ESO). Available from: https://doi.org/10.1093/eurheartj/ehae178

47. American Heart Association, 2025. Understanding blood pressure readings. Available from: https://www.heart.org/en/health-topics/high-blood-pressure/understanding-blood-pressure-readings

48. Ramzy I, 2019. Definition of hypertension and pressure goals during treatment (ESC-ESH Guidelines 2018). Available from: https://www.escardio.org/Journals/E-Journal-of-Cardiology-Practice/Volume-17/definition-of-hypertension-and-pressure-goals-during-treatment-esc-esh-guidelin

49. de Barcelos GT et al, 2022. Effects of aerobic training progression on blood pressure in individuals with hypertension: A systematic review with meta-analysis and meta-regression. Available from: https://www.ncbi.nlm.nih.gov/pmc/articles/PMC8891157/

50. Soltani S et al, 2020. Adherence to the dietary approaches to stop hypertension (DASH) diet in relation to all-cause and cause-specific mortality: a systematic review and dose-response meta-analysis of prospective cohort studies. Available from: https://doi.org/10.1186/s12937-020-00554-8

51. Neter JE et al, 2003. Influence of weight reduction on blood pressure. Available from: https://www.ahajournals.org/doi/10.1161/01.hyp.0000094221.86888.ae

52. Benjamim CJR et al, 2022. Nitrate derived from beetroot juice lowers bood pressure in patients with arterial hypertension: a systematic review and meta-analysis. Available from: https://www.ncbi.nlm.nih.gov/pmc/articles/PMC8965354/

53. Ried K, 2016. Garlic lowers blood pressure in hypertensive individuals, regulates serum cholesterol, and stimulates immunity: an updated meta-analysis and review. Available from: https://doi.org/10.3945/jn.114.202192

54. Herrera-Arellano A et al, 2004. Effectiveness and tolerability of a standardized extract from Hibiscus sabdariffa in patients with mild to moderate hypertension: a controlled and randomized clinical trial. Available from: https://www.sciencedirect.com/science/article/pii/S0944711304000029

55. Appleby PN et al, 2002. Hypertension and blood pressure among meat eaters, fish eaters, vegetarians and vegans in EPIC–Oxford. Available from: https://www.cambridge.org/core/journals/public-health-nutrition/article/hypertension-and-blood-pressure-among-meat-eaters-fish-eaters-vegetarians-and-vegans-in-epicoxford/678E54EF633FD623EF778BE1BA743C6A

56. Verma N et al, 2021. Non-pharmacological management of hypertension. Available from: https://www.ncbi.nlm.nih.gov/pmc/articles/PMC8678745/

57. CDC. Obesity and overweight. Available from: https://www.cdc.gov/nchs/fastats/obesity-overweight.htm

58. Office of Health Improvement and Disparities, 2024. Obesity profile: short statistical commentary May 2024. Available grom: https://www.gov.uk/government/statistics/update-to-the-obesity-profile-on-fingertips/obesity-profile-short-statistical-commentary-may-2024

59. Australian Institute of Health and Welfare, 2023. Overweight and obesity. Available from: https://www.aihw.gov.au/reports/overweight-obesity/overweight-and-obesity/contents/summary#health_impacts

60. Gielen M et al, 2018. Body mass index is negatively associated with telomere length: a collaborative cross-sectional meta-analysis of 87 observational studies. Available from: https://www.ncbi.nlm.nih.gov/pmc/articles/PMC6454526/

61. Wright N et al, 2017. The BROAD study: A randomised controlled trial using a whole food plant-based diet in the community for obesity, ischaemic heart disease or diabetes. Available from: https://www.nature.com/articles/nutd20173

62. Kannel W et al, 1996. Effect of weight on cardiovascular disease. Available from: https://www.sciencedirect.com/science/article/pii/S0002916523192264

63. Huang PL, 2009. A comprehensive definition for metabolic syndrome. Available from: https://doi.org/10.1242/dmm.001180

64. Pahwa R et al, 2023. Chronic inflammation. Available from: http://www.ncbi.nlm.nih.gov/books/NBK493173/

65. Xu B & Lin J, 2017. Characteristics and risk factors of rheumatoid arthritis in the United States: an NHANES analysis. Available from: https://www.ncbi.nlm.nih.gov/pmc/articles/PMC5703145/

66. Walrabenstein W et al, 2023. A multidisciplinary lifestyle program for rheumatoid arthritis: the 'Plants for Joints' randomized controlled trial. Available from: https://doi.org/10.1093/rheumatology/keac693

67. Chavez GN et al, 2023. The effects of plant-derived phytochemical compounds and phytochemical-rich diets on females with polycystic ovarian syndrome: a scoping review of clinical trials. Available from: https://www.mdpi.com/1660-4601/20/15/6534

68. Domínguez-López I et al, 2020. Effects of dietary phytoestrogens on hormones throughout a human lifespan: a review. Available from: https://www.mdpi.com/2072-6643/12/8/2456

69. McDougall R, 2012. NIH human microbiome project defines normal bacterial makeup of the body. Available from: https://www.nih.gov/news-events/news-releases/nih-human-microbiome-project-defines-normal-bacterial-makeup-body

70. Pistollato F et al, 2018. Nutritional patterns associated with the maintenance of neurocognitive functions and the risk of dementia and Alzheimer's disease: A focus on human studies. Available from: https://www.sciencedirect.com/science/article/pii/S1043661817316304

71. Okereke OI et al, 2012. Dietary fat types and 4-year cognitive change in community-dwelling older women. Available from: https://pubmed.ncbi.nih.gov/22605573/

72. Luukkonen PK et al, 2018. Saturated fat is more metabolically harmful to the human liver than unsaturated fat or simple sugars. Available from: https://www.ncbi.nih.gov/pmc/articles/PMC7082640

73. Venkatraman SK, 2018. Adverse effects on consumers health caused by hormones administered in cattle. Available from: researchgate.net/publication/339442430_ adverse_effects_on_consumers_health_ caused_by_hormones_administered_in_cattle

74. Mesfin YM et al, 2024. Veterinary drug residues in food products of animal origin and their public health consequences: A review. Available from: https://onlinelibrary.wiley.com/doi/abs/10.1002/vms3.70049

75. Zhuang P et al, 2021. Egg and cholesterol consumption and mortality from cardiovascular and different causes in the United States: A population cohort study. Available from: https://pubmed.ncbi.nlm.nih.gov/33561122/

76. Baker EA et al, 2006. The role of race and poverty in access to foods that enable individuals to adhere to dietary guidelines. Available from: https://www.ncbi.nlm.nih.gov/pmc/articles/PMC1636719/

77. Bevel MS et al, 2023. Association of food deserts and food swamps with obesity-related cancer mortality in the US. Available from: https://doi.org/10.1001/jamaoncol.2023.0634

78. Environmental Working Group, 2023. USDA livestock subsidies top $59 billion. Available from: https://www.ewg.org/news-insights/news/2023/08/usda-livestock-subsidies-top-59-billion.

79. Nahar L et al, 2020. Introduction of phytonutrients. Available from: https://doi.org/10.1007/978-981-13-1745-3_2-1

80. Panche AN et al, 2016. Flavonoids: an overview. Available from: https://www.ncbi.nlm.nih.gov/pmc/articles/PMC5465813/

81. Rodríguez-García C et al, 2019. Naturally lignan-rich foods: A dietary tool for health promotion? Available from: https://www.ncbi.nlm.nih.gov/pmc/articles/PMC6429205/

82. Consonni R & Ottolina G, 2022. NMR characterization of lignans. Available from: https://www.ncbi.nlm.nih.gov/pmc/articles/PMC9000441/

83. Kopylov AT et al, 2021. Diversity of plant sterols metabolism: The impact on human health, sport, and accumulation of contaminating sterols. Available from: https://www.ncbi.nlm.nih.gov/pmc/articles/PMC8150896/

84. Cleveland Clinic, What are adaptogens & types. Available from: https://my.clevelandclinic.org/health/drugs/22361-adaptogens
85. Office of Dietary Supplements, Vitamin D. Available from: https://ods.od.nih.gov/factsheets/VitaminD-HealthProfessional/
86. Muleya M et al, 2024. A comparison of the bioaccessible calcium supplies of various plant-based products relative to bovine milk. Available from: https://www.sciencedirect.com/science/article/pii/S0963996923013431
87. Office of Dietary Supplements—Vitamin C. Available from: https://ods.od.nih.gov/factsheets/VitaminC-HealthProfessional/
88. Febbraio MA & Karin M, 2021. "Sweet death": Fructose as a metabolic toxin that targets the gut-liver axis. Available from: https://www.cell.com/cell-metabolism/abstract/S1550-4131(21)00423-X
89. Annevelink C, 2023. Diet-derived and diet-related endogenously produced palmitic acid: Effects on metabolic regulation and cardiovascular disease risk. Available from: https://www.sciencedirect.com/science/article/pii/S1933287423002295
90. Shramko VS et al, 2020. The short overview on the relevance of fatty acids for human cardiovascular disorders. Available from: https://www.mdpi.com/2218-273X/10/8/1127
91. Monteiro CA et al, 2018. The UN decade of nutrition, the NOVA food classification and the trouble with ultra-processing. Available from: https://pubmed.ncbi.nlm.nih.gov/28322183/
92. European Commission, 2022. Goodbye E171: The EU bans titanium dioxide as a food additive. Available from: https://ec.europa.eu/newsroom/sante/items/732079/en
93. Topiwala A et al, 2017. Moderate alcohol consumption as risk factor for adverse brain outcomes and cognitive decline: longitudinal cohort study. Available from: https://www.bmj.com/content/357/bmj.j2353
94. World Health Organization, 2023. Sodium reduction. Available from: https://www.who.int/news-room/fact-sheets/detail/salt-reduction
95. Feng Q et al, 2024. Waist-to-height ratio and body fat percentage as risk factors for ischemic cardiovascular disease: A prospective cohort study from UK Biobank. Available from: https://ajcn.nutrition.org/article/S0002-9165(24)00388-5/fulltext
96. Gearhardt AN & DiFeliceantonio AG, 2023. Highly processed foods can be considered addictive substances based on established scientific criteria. Available from: https://onlinelibrary.wiley.com/doi/abs/10.1111/add.16065

97. U.S. Department of Agriculture and U.S. Department of & Health and Human Services, 2020. Dietary guidelines for Americans, 2020-2025, 9th Edition. Available from: https://www.dietaryguidelines.gov/resources/2020-2025-dietary-guidelines-online-materials

98. CDC, 2022. Sugar sweetened beverage intake. Available from: https://www.cdc.gov/nutrition/data-statistics/sugar-sweetened-beverages-intake.html

99. Escobar Gil T & Laverde Gil J, 2023. Artificially sweetened beverages beyond the metabolic risks: A systematic review of the literature. Available from: https://www.ncbi.nlm.nih.gov/pmc/articles/PMC9891650/

100. USDA, 2005. Overview of food additives. Available from: https://www.ams.usda.gov/sites/default/files/media/flavors%20nonsynthetic%202%20TR.pdf

101. FoodData Central, Kale. Available from: https://fdc.nal.usda.gov/fdc-app.html#/food-details/323505/nutrients

102. McColl K, Increasing fruit and vegetable consumption to reduce the risk of noncommunicable diseases. Available from: https://www.who.int/tools/elena/commentary/fruit-vegetables-ncds

103. Slavin J, 2003. Why whole grains are protective: biological mechanisms. Available from: https://www.cambridge.org/core/journals/proceedings-of-the-nutrition-society/article/why-whole-grains-are-protective-biological-mechanisms/25042F202584EDAE68C7CBBFCDBB5471

104. Hollænder PL et al, 2015. Whole-grain and blood lipid changes in apparently healthy adults: a systematic review and meta-analysis of randomized controlled studies. Available from: https://www.sciencedirect.com/science/article/pii/S0002916523126955

105. Ghanbari-Gohari F et al, 2022. Consumption of whole grains and risk of type 2 diabetes: A comprehensive systematic review and dose-response meta-analysis of prospective cohort studies. Available from: https://onlinelibrary.wiley.com/doi/abs/10.1002/fsn3.2811

106. Dholariya SJ & Orrick JA, 2024. Biochemistry, fructose metabolism. Available from: http://www.ncbi.nlm.nih.gov/books/NBK576428/

107. DeChristopher LR et al, 2020. High fructose corn syrup, excess-free-fructose, and risk of coronary heart disease among African Americans–the Jackson Heart Study. Available from: https://doi.org/10.1186/s40795-020-00396-x

108. Meli R et al, 2020. Oxidative stress and BPA toxicity: An antioxidant approach for male and female reproductive dysfunction. Available from: https://www.mdpi.com/2076-3921/9/5/405

109. Lopez MJ & Mohiuddin SS, 2024. Biochemistry, essential amino acids. Available from: http://www.ncbi.nlm.nih.gov/books/NBK557845/

110. Bolland MJ et al, 2015. Calcium intake and risk of fracture: systematic review. Available from: https://pubmed.ncbi.nlm.nih.gov/26420387/

111. Fallon Nevada: FAQs: Organophosphates CDC Archive. Available from: https://archive.cdc.gov/#/details?url=https://www.cd.c.gov/nceh/clusters/Fallon/organophosfaq.htm

112. FDA, 2024. GMO crops, animal food, and beyond. Available from: https://www.fda.gov/food/agricultural-biotechnology/gmo-crops-animal-food-and-beyond

113. Jach ME & Serefko A, 2018. Chapter 9—nutritional yeast biomass: characterization and application. Available from: https://www.sciencedirect.com/science/article/pii/B9780128114407000090

114. TatahMentan M et al, 2020. Toxic and essential elements in rice and other grains from the United States and other countries. Available from: https://www.mdpi.com/1660-4601/17/21/8128

115. Food Standards Agency. Review of methods for the analysis of culinary herbs and spices for authenticity. Available from: https://www.food.gov.uk/research/research-projects/review-of-methods-for-the-analysis-of-culinary-herbs-and-spices-for-authenticity

116. Vicennati V et al, 2009. Stress-related development of obesity and cortisol in women. Available from: https://onlinelibrary.wiley.com/doi/abs/10.1038/oby.2009.76

117. Shetty AK et al, 2018. Emerging anti-aging strategies-scientific basis and efficacy. Available from: https://www.aginganddisease.org/EN/10.14336/AD.2018.1026

118. Barnard ND et al, 2023. A dietary intervention for vasomotor symptoms of menopause: a randomized, controlled trial. Available from: https://journals.lww.com/menopausejournal/fulltext/2023/01000/a_dietary_intervention_for_vasomotor_symptoms_of.12.aspx

119. Sims S & Yeager S, 2022. Next level: Your guide to kicking ass, feeling great, and crushing goals through menopause and beyond. Available from: https://amzn.to/4jEu6FA

120. Haver MC, 2024. The new menopause: Navigating your path through hormonal change with purpose, power, and facts. Available from: https://amzn.to/4jEu6FA

Resources

All the resources on these pages are available at my website https://fabuloushealthbook.net/resources.

For more information on the health benefits of a whole plant foods diet, I highly recommend the following organisations. The information is free, but as non-profit organisations, you can support them by donation.

Physician's Commission for Responsible Medicine *pcrm.org*

Nutrition Facts *nutritionfacts.org*

T Colin Campbell Center for Nutrition Studies *nutritionstudies.org*

Plantbased Health Professions (UK) *plantbasedhealthprofessionals.com*

Plant Based Health Australia *wholefoodsplantbasedhealth.com.au*

Plants For Health (NL) *plants-for-health.com*

Chapter 3:

QUIT line *1-800-QUIT-NOW*

Alcoholics Anonymous *aa.org*

Chapter 4:

Ornish lifestyle medicine *ornish.com*

Chapter 12:

Nutrition labels

accessdata.fda.gov/scripts/InteractiveNutritionFactsLabel/default.cfm

Chapter 15:

Sweet Indulgence Desserts by Chef AJ *amzn.to/41smf7R*

Meal Planner *fabuloushealthbook.net/bonuses*

Chapter 19:

Well Your World Veggie Broth Mix *wellyourworld.com/?aff=29*

Butler Soy Curls *amzn.to/4faWq0a*

Epic Vegan! By Dustin Harder *amzn.to/3BWsGFV*

Epic Vegan Quick and Easy by Dustin Harder *amzn.to/3NxeAgK*

JOI plant milk bases *addjoi.com/fabuloushealth*

Use the code FABULOUSHEALTH for 10% off.

Chapter 20:

James Clear—Atomic Habits Book *amzn.to/48mtYWH*

James Clear—Atomic Habits Audible *amzn.to/3NyLWfh*

Audible FREE TRIAL *amzn.to/3C4iNFX*

Chapter 21:

Great plant-based movies *fabuloushealth.net/resources*

Chapter 23:

Facebook Group *facebook.com/groups/wfpblifestyleforbeginners*

By using the links above I may receive a small commission from the supplier. Thank you for supporting my work to help you become healthier. Not all of the links are income generating.

Thank you for reading Fabulous Health: A Simple Plan To Get Well And Stay Well.

I appreciate you and wish for you a life of Fabulous Health.

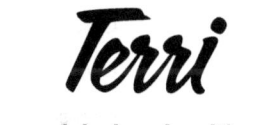

www.fabuloushealth.net

Index

A

Adaptogens 84
Ad libitum 235
Aging 62, 64
Air fryer 155
Alcohol 47, 79, 94
Alzheimer's disease 30, 42, 53
Amino acids 80, 134, 168
Angina 55
Animal products 49, 51, 54, 64, 67, 91, 152
Anthocyanins 66, 84
Anthropometric measurements 101
Antinutrients 85
Antioxidants 50, 65, 81, 83, 122
Appendix 271
Arrabiata 253
ASOUPAS 91
Atherosclerosis 54, 84, 93, 234
Autoimmune disease 65

B

Bean Burgers 261
Beans 120, 126, 172, 260
Bechamel 259
Behavior change 203
Bibliography 272
Bioimpedance 102
Biometric measurements 101
Biotin 137
Black bean and tempeh casserole 260

Blender 154
Bliss point 72
Blood pressure 56, 58, 63, 66, 100, 109, 125, 234, 241
Blood tests 99
Body fat calculation 103
Body measurements 100
Bread 124
Breakfast 135, 185, 186, 225, 247
Breast cancer 48
Budget 171
Bulk 142, 159, 173
Butter Beans 262

C

Cake 212
Calcium 83, 86, 87, 136, 196
Cancer 29, 47, 50, 61, 65
Carbohydrates 79, 80, 92, 150
Cardiovascular disease 49, 63, 64, 67, 83, 87, 93, 105, 115, 122, 236
Carotenoids 83
Celiac disease 138
Checkups 241
Cheese 167, 195, 196
Cheezy Sauce 263
Chia and banana pudding 269
Chili 127, 174, 255
Chloride 83
Chocolate mousse 268
Cholesterol 53, 54, 99, 149
Clean fifteen 159
Cobalamin 137
Coffee 120, 127

Community 229

Condiments 126, 129

Connection to others 42

Conventional produce 157

Cookies 267

Coronary artery disease 55

C-reactive protein 100, 233

Crohn's disease 67

Cupcakes 166

D

Dairy 48, 113, 164

Date Snickers 269

Dementia 42, 55, 56, 61, 72, 87, 94

DEXA 101

Diabetes 39, 41, 49, 51, 52, 53, 61, 64

Dietary guidelines 39, 74

Dinner 226, 253

Dirty dozen 158

DNA 47, 50, 62, 80, 83, 136, 137

Drive-through 114

Dyslipidemia 53, 63

E

Energy density 119, 186

Environment 64, 73, 113

Environmental working group 158

Exercise 39, 47, 58, 61, 201, 242

F

Fasting glucose 100

Fat 51, 81, 149

Fiber 50, 64, 122, 126, 172, 236

Flavonoids 84

Flour 124

Folate 137

Food desert 73

Food label 147, 148

Food processor 154

Freezer 174, 181

Fries 166, 212

Fruit 120, 125, 129, 171, 248

G

Gelato 270

Gestational diabetes 52

Gluten-free 138

Goal setting 107

Government subsidies 75

Granola 212, 247

Greens 50, 59, 79, 87

Green Smoothie 251

Gut 64, 67, 68, 137, 138

H

Habits 201

Hashimoto's 65

HbA1c 52, 66, 99, 109, 241

Healthy foods 128

Heart disease 53, 54, 55, 56, 61, 72, 73, 84, 86, 92, 95, 105, 116, 125, 218

Height 101

Herbs 120, 126, 172

Hibiscus tea 59

High fructose 92

High fructose corn syrup 92, 125, 147

Holidays 228

Hormones 65, 126, 134, 136, 196

Hummus 212, 266

Hypertension 56, 57, 63

I

Inflammation 64

Ingredients 147

Instant pot 154

Insulin resistance 63

Intermittent fasting 236

Iodine 83

Irritable bowel syndrome 68

J

Journal 110

Juicing 236

Junk food 113, 165

K

Knives 153

L

Lasagna 258

Legumes 120, 126, 129

Lignans 84

Living with others 115

Lunch 135, 175, 187, 226, 253

M

Mac'n'cheeze 264

Macronutrients 79

Magnesium 83

Marketing 74

Mash 257

Mayo 265

Meal planning 182

Meat 48, 113, 194

Medications 241

Menopause 242

Metabolic syndrome 63

Micronutrients 81

Microwave 155

Minerals 82

Minestrone 254

Multivitamins 88

Mushroom gravy 266

N

Navy method 102

Negative people 229

Niacin 136

Ninja strategy 142

Nutrient density 119

Nutritional yeast 168

Nuts 127

O

Obesity 47, 61, 62, 64, 72, 92, 115, 218

Oil 93, 113, 168

Omega 3 87

Organic 157

Oven 155

P

Pancakes 252

Pantothenic Acid 136

Pantry staples 173

Parmesan 196, 258

Parties 227

Pasta Sauce 253

PCOS 66

Peer pressure 229

Perfection 213

Phosphorus 83

Photos 105

Physical activity 39

Phytonutrients 81, 83

Plant-based 39, 66, 67, 75, 164

Plant-based cheese 167

Plant-based meat alternatives 167

Plant Milk 196

Plant sterols 84

Plateau 233

Potassium 83

Pots and pans 154

Prepping 179

Protein 80, 134, 150

Protein powder 135

Purple Smoothie 251

Puttanesca 254

Pyridoxine 137

Q

Queso 195

Quiz Answers 271

R

Reproduction problems 66

Resources 282

Restaurants 226

Rheumatoid arthritis 65

Riboflavin 136

Ricotta 195, 264

Risky behaviors 41

Risotto 256

S

Salad 187, 188

Salt 58, 95

Saturated fat 53, 54, 55, 72, 81, 93

Scale 104, 220

Scrambled tofu 250

Seeds 127

Selenium 83

Self-doubt 217

Serving size 149

Shepherd's pie 257

Sigh 235

Sleep 41

SMART goals 107, 108

Smoking 41

Smoothie 236, 237, 251

Smoothie bowls 167

Snacks 181, 267

Soda 115

Sodium 83, 150

Soup 174, 175

Soy 49, 249

Soy curls 174

Spaghetti 174, 194

Spices 120, 126, 172

Stress 40, 60

Sugar 92, 150

Sugar-free 120

Sugar-free soda 116

Supplements 85

Swaps 132, 193, 207

T

Taco 194

Tea 120

Tempeh 195, 260

The 100% rule 208

Thiamin 136

Tofu 174, 195, 250, 259, 264, 268

Transitional food 163

Transitioning 207

Travel 225

Triglycerides 63, 99

Type 1 diabetes 52

Type 2 diabetes 51

U

Ulcerative colitis 67

Ultra-processed food 49, 93, 113

USDA guidelines 74

V

Vegan 165

Vegetable chopper 153

Vegetables 120, 122, 129, 171

Veggies for breakfast 185

Visceral adiposity 63

Vitamin B12 85, 100

Vitamin C 88

Vitamin D 86, 100

Vitamins 82, 136

W

Waist-to-hip ratio 104

Weight 100, 220

Weight loss 109

Whole grains 120, 123, 129, 172

Y

Yogurt 212, 249

Z

Zinc 83

www.ingramcontent.com/pod-product-compliance
Lightning Source LLC
Chambersburg PA
CBHW060453030426
42337CB00015B/1573